T0201894

Working Alliance Skills for Mental Health Professionals

Working Alliance Skills for Mental Health Professionals

Edited by

JAIRO N. FUERTES

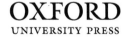

OXFORD
UNIVERSITY PRESS

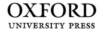

OXFORD
UNIVERSITY PRESS

Oxford University Press is a department of the University of Oxford. It furthers
the University's objective of excellence in research, scholarship, and education
by publishing worldwide. Oxford is a registered trade mark of Oxford University
Press in the UK and certain other countries.

Published in the United States of America by Oxford University Press
198 Madison Avenue, New York, NY 10016, United States of America.

CIP data is on file at the Library of Congress
ISBN 978-0-19-086852-9

To my wife Hnin, and to my daughters, Sofia and Isabella. A special dedication to my mother, Esther, and to my father, Pedro Pablo Fuertes (1936–2018).

Contents

Preface

The impetus for this book comes from years of teaching and supervising graduate-level students and my being asked by thoughtful students some variation of the following question: "How do I go about establishing the working alliance?" In this volume, we focus on the working alliance, specifically Bordin's (1979) conceptualization of the working alliance, which emphasizes therapist–client agreement on the goals and tasks of treatment and the existence of an emotional bond between the two participants. A perusal of the literature on the working alliance revealed that hundreds of studies have been conducted on this specific conceptualization. Given the popularity of the concept of the working alliance and the considerable research that has been conducted about it, it is surprising to find that there is little published work about the skills that are used in sessions to establish and sustain the working alliance. To address this gap in the literature, in this book the authors provide examples of in-session therapist interventions and behaviors that can guide you in ways to establish and sustain the working alliance.

In the psychological literature, the working alliance between a clinician and a patient is considered a *sine qua non* of successful treatment (Lambert & Barley, 2001). Hundreds of studies in the field of psychotherapy have consistently shown that the working alliance is the strongest and most consistent predictor of outcome in treatment (Norcross & Lambert, 2018). Given this evidence from empirical studies, this seems like an optimal time to prepare a book that helps students who have questions about the mechanics of establishing and maintaining a working alliance. Currently, trainees rely on supervisors who may or may not be in a position to demonstrate such skills or may not be able to communicate how to form effective alliances. This book should be helpful to students in courses that teach relationship-building skills and courses that focus on helping skills. I also hope that the book will be helpful to students from a variety of mental healthcare–providing disciplines (e.g., counselor educators, social work) and to new professionals and even seasoned teachers, clinicians, and supervisors who are interested in the working alliance. In many of the chapters, the authors define each dimension of the working alliance and describe the specific mechanisms and interventions that the provider can use to establish and sustain it. We provide examples and ways that the reader can practice these skills, and provide the relevant empirical evidence for each topic discussed. However, this volume does *not* contain a complete review of the literature in each area.

As editor, I specifically asked the authors to cite just enough literature to support the content presented, but also to rely on their years of clinical, supervisory, and teaching experience and wisdom in presenting the skills. There are other volumes containing exhaustive reviews of research on the working alliance, most notably as of this writing Norcross's *Therapy Relationships that Work*, also published by Oxford University Press.

In setting parameters for the book chapters, it seemed important to identify the different areas of possible relevance to the reader and to select the ones that seemed to be most important. After I selected these areas, I then contacted authors about contributing to the volume. Once they agreed to contribute chapters based on their expertise and experience in teaching and writing about the working alliance, I sent them parameters to guide them in their work. These parameters noted the emphasis on clinical application and the presentation of the most relevant skills (i.e., in-session interventions and behaviors) in each area. Authors were reminded that the book is anchored by Bordin's (1979) pantheoretical conceptualization of the working alliance, comprising agreement on goals, tasks, and the development of a bond between therapist and client. They were provided the definition of the working alliance offered by Gelso and Carter (1994); that is, the alignment of the reasonable self/ego of the client with the working or "therapizing" ego of the therapist in order for work to take place. They were told that, as per Gelso and others, techniques are not seen as the alliance per se, but that the alliance is comprised of a sense of shared mission, of being on the same side or page, and of feeling a sense of consensus and/or collaboration. I shared that, in my view, therapist skills (i.e., in-session interventions and behaviors) contribute to the development of the working alliance—that sense of collaboration and trust between therapist and client.

Authors were further reminded that the book is intended for graduate students early in training in master's and doctoral level counseling and clinical programs, so that they can learn and put to use clinical skills to help them develop and nurture the working alliance. However, they were also told that the book might also be of value to early career professionals and even seasoned clinicians. I asked them to keep a developmental perspective in presenting the material: start with what seems basic and then present material that may be more challenging or advanced. They were instructed to include the relevant theoretical literature and the empirical evidence (when it exists) for the skills highlighted, but to include just enough to make the case since the core of the chapter should be on demonstrating with examples how the skills that seem most essential and salient can be put to use. I asked authors to rely on their teaching and clinical experience and wisdom as a valuable contribution to the chapter and to trust their judgment as they think about clinical scenarios and as they developed clinical examples. They were asked to keep in mind, where possible, that the focus is on maintaining and sustaining the working alliance, and, therefore, to note if the skills presented were more appropriate for establishing an alliance (i.e., in the first session, certainly within the first three sessions of therapy), or to note if other skills may come into play later in therapy in sustaining the alliance. I also asked them, where and when possible, to note how the working alliance skills highlighted are informed by the three broad schools of psychotherapy: psychoanalytic/psychodynamic, cognitive-behavioral, and humanistic/existential. Finally, I reminded them that the focus of the chapter should be on individual psychotherapy with adults. I believe that the authors diligently followed these broad parameters and that the result is a set of easy to read yet clinically useful chapters that will help you understand the mechanics of Bordin's working alliance concept. This book will help you, along with the rest of your training, to be a more effective therapist.

I am grateful to the authors who have contributed chapters to the book. The reader can be sure that they are all trusted scholars and seasoned teachers and clinicians who have thought about this topic for many years. To all of them, I extend my deepest gratitude.

References

Bordin, E. S. (1979). The generalizability of the psychoanalytic concept of the working alliance. *Psychotherapy: Theory, Research & Practice, 16*(3), 252–260. http://dx.doi.org/10.1037/h0085885.

Gelso, C. J., & Carter, J. A. (1994). Components of the psychotherapy relationship: Their interaction and unfolding during treatment. *Journal of Counseling Psychology, 41*(3), 296–306. http://dx.doi.org/10.1037/0022-0167.41.3.296.

Lambert, M. J., & Barley, D. E. (2001). Research summary on the therapeutic relationship and psychotherapy outcome. *Psychotherapy: Theory, Research, Practice, Training, 38*(4), 357–361. http://dx.doi.org/10.1037/0033-3204.38.4.357.

Norcoss, J. C., & Lambert, M. J. (2018). Psychotherapy relationships that work III. *Psychotherapy, 55,* 303–315.

Acknowledgments

I am grateful to the Gordon F. Derner School of Psychology and to Adelphi University for providing me with a sabbatical leave to work on this book. I would also like to thank the following colleagues for their valuable contributions in reading and commenting on previous drafts of some of the chapters: Charles J. Gelso, Aaiza Naumann, Mariela Reyes, and Patrick Mele.

List of Contributors

Timothy Anderson, PhD
Professor
Department of Psychology
Ohio University
Athens, Ohio, USA

Robinder Bedi, PhD
Associate Professor
Educational and Counselling Psychology
  and Special Education
University of British Columbia
Vancouver, BC, Canada

Changming Duan, PhD
Professor
Educational Psychology
University of Kansas
Lawrence, KS, United States

Catherine F. Eubanks, PhD
Associate Professor
Ferkauf Graduate School of Psychology
Yeshiva University
Bronx, NY, USA

Jairo N. Fuertes, PhD, ABPP, LMHC
Professor of Psychology
Gordon F Derner School of Psychology
Adelphi University
Garden City, NY, USA

Jerald Gardner, PhD
Assistant Clinical Professor
Psychiatry
Mount Sinai Beth Israel
New York, NY, USA

Jazmin M. González, MEd
Doctoral Student
Counseling and Educational Psychology
New Mexico State University
Las Cruces, New Mexico, USA

Rodney K. Goodyear, PhD
Professor
Counseling and Human Services
University of Redlands
Redlands, California, US

Lauren Lipner, MA
Doctoral Candidate
Psychology
Adelphi University
Garden City, NY, USA

Patrick Mele, MA
Research Assistant
Derner School of Psychology
Adelphi University
Garden City, New York, USA

Michael Moore
Gordon F. Derner School of Psychology
Adelphi University
Garden City, NY, USA

J. Christopher Muran, PhD
Associate Dean & Full Professor: Director
Gordon F. Derner School of Psychology;
  Psychotherapy Research Program
Adelphi University; Mount Sinai
  Beth Israel
Garden City; New York, NY, USA

Chloe Pagano-Stalzer, MA
Doctoral Candidate
Clinical Psychology
Derner School of Psychology at
    Adelphi University
Garden City, New York, United States
    of America

Matthew Perlman, MS
Graduate Student
Psychology
Ohio University
Athens, OH, USA

Andres Perez-Rojas, PhD
Assistant Professor
Counseling and Educational Psychology
New Mexico State University
Las Cruces, NM, United States

Julian Rapaport, MA
Doctoral Student
Clinical Psychology
Adelphi University
Garden City, NY, USA

Hideko Sera, PsyD
Associate Dean
Clinical Psychology
School of Education
University of Redlands
Redlands, California, USA

Georgiana Shick Tryon, PhD
Professor Emerita
Ph.D. Program in Educational
    Psychology
The Graduate Center, CUNY
City, New York, USA

1

Working Alliance Skills
for Healthcare Professionals

Introduction

Jairo N. Fuertes, Patrick Mele, and Julian Rapaport

Sigmund Freud's genius provided the basis for what we all know today as psychotherapy. While alternative and viable forms of psychoanalysis and psychotherapy have been developed since his time, Freud has figured in some way, shape, or form as either the impetus for the advancement and refinement of what he originally proposed or, in many cases, as a complete departure from his ideas and method. In the case of the working alliance, it is no different. Freud discovered a method for helping patients suffering from psychological distress, and this method inevitably involved a patient and a doctor meeting and collaborating together for the purpose of alleviating psychological discomfort and pain. Freud never used the terms "alliance" or "working alliance," but he clearly pointed to the importance of patience and collaboration—and a great deal of dedication on the part of both the patient and the analyst in helping the patient experience relief of problematic symptoms. In his theoretical considerations, Freud (1912/1990) shifted from seeing the patient's experience and relationship with the therapist as inevitably neurotic, based on troubling unconscious material that relied on the defensive mechanism of projection, to a view that allowed for the benefits of positive transference, or unconscious positive feelings, of the patient for the doctor. In later writings, Freud seemed to have adjusted his views even further to allow for the possibility that the patient and the doctor could establish a connection based on conscious nonconflictual thoughts and feelings, where the participants could have reality-based perceptions of one another. Freud's views of progress and healing in treatment still placed a great emphasis on the interpretation of the troubling unconscious feelings and experiences for the patient but subsequently allowed for the possibility that healing also involved the patient's nonpathological perceptions and conscious exchanges with the therapist.

Sterba's (1940) early psychoanalytic conceptualization benefitted from innovations made in ego psychology and further advanced the notion that although the patient's experience in treatment involved transference and distortion, the patient brought to treatment valuable knowledge of him- or herself and past personal experiences which greatly aided the therapist's work in treatment. Sterba expanded the idea that successful treatment involved a partnership between the patient's reasonable self emerging in therapy and working in tandem with the therapist toward psychological growth. A short time later and consistent with the evolution in thought within psychoanalysis toward a two-person, object relations perspective, Elizabeth Zetzel (1956) conceptualized the relationship between patient and analyst as a "therapeutic alliance," arguing that one could differentiate transference not just as neurosis/resistance but also as a "therapeutic alliance" that emerged from the patient's "mature ego functions." The concept of the therapeutic alliance was considerably elevated and renamed the "working alliance" by Ralph Greenson (1967). Greenson's conceptualization of the working alliance accounted for the patient's efforts and arduous work in having, on the one hand, to experience and express the painful and regressive ideas that emerged in treatment from free association and, on the other hand, to endure the demands of analysis. Greenson further proposed that the patient in analysis was capable of developing a nonsexualized and nonaggressive relationship with the analyst, one that was crucial to the work in treatment, and that this capacity stemmed from the patient having had these types of relationships in the past. Greenson also humanizes the therapist and points to the qualities of the analyst which make the working alliance possible; namely, the balance between objective attention and analysis of the content brought up by the patient and a therapeutic stance that is "compassionate, empathic, straightforward, and non-judgmental" (p. 46).

Bordin (1979) generalized what was largely a psychoanalytic concept and offered an operationalization of the working alliance that he believed to be pantheoretical (i.e., it provided a view of the working alliance as it emerges in all psychological treatments). Given the vast numbers of therapies that were emerging in his lifetime, Bordin also intended his conceptualization of the working alliance to provide convergence in theory and research. Bordin proposed that the working alliance could be conceived of and measured in terms of three distinct components: the extent to which the client and therapist agree on the goals and tasks of treatment (regardless of whether these are implicit or explicit) and the extent to which there is an emerging bond between them, characterized by trust. Bordin's conceptualization altered the way that we view the working alliance in therapy. He extracted from it the psychoanalytic qualities of transference, of the unconscious, and the unique role of the analyst as the interpreter of reality. Bordin's conception of the working alliance provided much more value to the role of the client and the therapist in actively collaborating and achieving some sense of agreement or consensus about the nature of treatment. As noted in the Preface, the focus of this book is on the skills associated with building and sustaining the working alliance as conceptualized by Bordin.

A considerable amount of conceptual work has been directed at mapping the working alliance within the broader therapy relationship and also within the overall process of therapy. Gelso and Carter (1985, 1994), building on the work of Greenson (1967), suggested that all psychotherapy relationships consist of three components: a working alliance, a real relationship, and a transference configuration, and they hypothesized that these components exist in all forms of counseling and psychotherapy, not just psychoanalysis. In their "tripartite" conceptualization of the relationship in therapy, Gelso and Carter (1985, 1994) conceived of the working alliance as the more contractual and purposive aspect of the interactions between the provider and client, comprised of goals, tasks, and trust, following Bordin's original definition. They proposed that the real relationship is defined as the more personal, or person-to-person relationship between the provider and the client, where the goals and purpose of the treatment fade into the background and the personal qualities of each human being surface in the interactions. The real relationship involves more personal perceptions, such as whether one likes the other, feels connected, and can be relaxed and who they are in the interaction. The components of the real relationship, according to Gelso (2002, 2011) are genuineness, realism, magnitude, and valence.

The third dimension of the relationship is the transference/countertransference configuration, which deals with more "neurotic" aspects of relating in treatment, including projection and the displacement of past unresolved conflicts or current unresolved problems onto the other in the relationship. While the transference/countertransference dynamic has been theorized about and discussed the longest, and major theoretical developments have been advanced since Freud, it has received relatively little empirical attention. This is due perhaps to the elusive nature of the concept and the difficulties in operationalizing these constructs in research. Nonetheless, some research has been conducted in the past couple of decades (Fuertes, Gelso, Owen, & Cheng, 2015). The real relationship is the most recent construct, and, with the recent publication of measures for use with therapists and clients, research activity on this construct has increased substantially (Gelso, Kivlighan, & Markin, 2018).

In contrast to the limited empirical attention that the real relationship has received (see Gelso, Kivlighan, & Making, 2018, for a recent review) and the scarce empirical attention on transference/countertransference (see Hayes, Gelso, Goldberg, & Kivlighan, 2018, for a recent review of countertransference management), the working alliance has been an integral part of the psychotherapy research literature for decades. Horvath and colleagues (2011) conducted a search for the electronic literature on the alliance; that search generated more than 7,000 articles. One factor that is responsible for the continued interest in the alliance is the consistent finding of a significant positive relationship between stronger alliances and psychotherapy treatment outcomes (Lambert & Barley, 2001). Horvath (2001) conducted a meta-analysis based on their search and selected 190 independent studies that examined the relationship between alliance and outcome; they found a significant effect size ($r = 0.275$, $p < 0.001$), a finding consistent with previous studies (e.g., Horvath & Bedi, 2002). Flückiger, Del Re, Wampold, and Horvath (2018) conducted the most recent meta-analysis of the alliance with adult patients and examined its link with outcome. Their analyses included 295 studies and more than 30,000 patients, and again, consistent with previous meta-analyses, they found effects sizes in the range of .25 to .29. These results have provided irrefutable evidence of the relationship between alliance and outcome and include consistent findings that show that the connection between stronger alliances and better treatment outcomes is robust and is not influenced by therapeutic modality, treatment length, or the number of participants involved in each study. While different assessments of alliance have been used in the empirical research, Flückiger et al. found no significant differences in the alliance–outcome relationship, whether the alliance was measured as Bordin's working alliance or via alternative conceptualizations (see Chapter 5).

To examine the variability of scores on the working alliance, we reviewed 17 articles from the meta-analysis conducted by Flückiger, Del Re, Wampold, and Horvath (2018) to evaluate the range of alliance scores in individual adult psychotherapy. All 17 studies utilized a version of the Working Alliance Inventory (WAI) and included 1,407 clients/patients and 26 therapists. For clients, the range of observed alliance total scores was between 149.7 (4.15) and 237.3 (6.59), with an average of 200.46 (5.57). The score in parenthesis is the scale score on the WAI, which has a range of 1–7, where a higher score indicates a stronger working alliance. For therapists, the range of observed alliance scores was between 185.94 (5.16) and 208.16 (5.78), with an average of 198.04 (5.50). This analysis indicates that clients tend to have a wider range of experiences of the working alliance than therapists (4.15 is a rating slightly above "sometimes" and 6.59 is a rating between "very often" and "always" on the WAI scale). For therapists, 5.16 is a score slightly above "often" and 5.78 is closer to "very often." The average working alliance score for clients and therapists is almost identical (5.57 and 5.50, respectively, right between "often" and "very often"). To account for the possibility that their findings were due to bias from the current lot of published studies, Flückiger et al. (2018) reported that more than a thousand additional unpublished studies would have to be found in order to significantly reduce the effect sizes that they uncovered.

Although the effect sizes found for the relationship between alliance and outcome have been small to moderate, this still represents a sizeable and consistent finding due to the complexity of the variable in question—psychotherapy (Castonguay, Constantino, & Holtforth, 2006; Horvath et al., 2011). Overall, the alliance has become known as a "common factor" or "process of change" in psychotherapy research, and a better alliance represents one of the strongest predictors of treatment success in the current research literature (Castonguay et al., 2006). As Lambert and Barley (2001) aptly stated, "The improvement of psychotherapy may best be accomplished by learning to improve one's ability to relate to clients and tailoring that relationship to individual clients" (p. 357).

Despite the "settled science" linking working alliance to outcome, there has been very little writing about the skills that are inherent in developing and sustaining the working alliance. Current research indicates that formal alliance training in psychology graduate schools is minimal. A study conducted by Constantino, Morrison, Coyne, and Howard (2017) recruited 305 directors of clinical training (DCTs) across the United States and Canada (236 affiliated with American Psychological Association [APA]-accredited clinical and psychology graduate programs) and surveyed them on several alliance training domains. The results of their survey showed that, generally, programs have not systematically incorporated formal alliance training, although the majority of DCTs agreed that formal alliance training elements should be incorporated into their curricula (Constantino et al., 2017). In addition, Levendosky and Hopwood (2016) noted that although there is abundant evidence that the working alliance is associated with treatment outcomes and that the alliance is accepted as a mechanism for change across therapeutic modalities, formal working alliance training has been largely neglected.

The need to develop training programs that specifically focus on the working alliance fits with the positions from Divisions 12 (Clinical), 17 (Counseling), and 29 (Psychotherapy) of the APA. According to the Standards of Accreditation for Health Service Psychology published by the APA in 2015, psychology doctoral students and interns are expected to "establish and maintain effective therapeutic relationships, develop evidence-based treatment plans specific to the service delivery goals, and implement interventions informed by the current scientific literature, assessment findings, diversity characteristics, and contextual variables." Additionally, the APA's Recognition of Psychotherapy Effectiveness clearly states that "psychotherapy is rooted and enhanced by a therapeutic alliance between therapist and client/patient" (APA, 2012). The working alliance has been shown to help cultivate and sustain therapeutic relationships with patients/clients and to bring in the perspective of the patient/client by emphasizing consensus and collaboration. Therefore, incorporating formal working alliance training into graduate psychology curricula is not only beneficial, but also a necessity for fulfilling the APA requirements for accreditation.

It is evident that there is broad consensus that the working alliance is a critical tool of successful psychotherapy and that graduate students should formally learn how to develop the necessary skills for establishing and maintaining a good working alliance. However, as Constantino et al. (2017) note from their survey study, there is a "disconnect between what clinical faculty are aware of and regard as important training principles, and what is being done to train clinical students in best alliance practices" (Constantino et al., 2017). Addressing this disconnect is a goal of the current volume. While we do not present a training program per se, the chapters do address some of the fundamental skill sets that the authors considered as most important in establishing and sustaining the working alliance, and this may be an important first step in developing a working alliance training program.

Our preceding analysis of the range of working alliance scores, as well as the average ratings reported by clients and therapists, indicated relatively high scores, even though formal working alliance training has not been implemented in graduate training. It is quite likely that current training that includes achieving proficiency in helping skills, skill in establishing Rogerian core conditions in sessions such as conveying empathy and "prizing" the client, and proficiency in the technical and conceptual aspects of various approaches to therapy give trainees a great deal to work with in developing the working alliance. However, that is not to say that formal training will not improve working alliance experiences for clients (and therapists) and increase the modest to moderate link between the working alliance and clinical outcome. It is possible that even a modest statistical increase in variance explained in outcome, obtained via explicit/formal working alliance training/practice, may translate into clinically meaningful change.

The layout of the book is such that it covers the essential dimensions of the working alliance as conceptualized by Bordin. In Chapter 2, entitled "The Bond of the Working Alliance," the authors describe and discuss the "working bond" aspect of Bordin's conceptualization of the working alliance. Within the working alliance, the bond refers to an emotional attachment formed and maintained between client/patient and therapist. This bond reflects the feelings and attitudes that client/patient and therapist have toward each other and enables the therapeutic work through a sense of collaboration and trust. First, the authors discuss the defining features of the bond. Then, they identify various skills and facilitative attitudes that can foster the bond, such as empathy, unconditional positive regard, and genuineness. Finally, they discuss how the working bond and possible ruptures will manifest at various stages in the treatment, from building the initial bond to working through termination. In Chapter 3, entitled "Therapeutic Interpersonal Skills for Facilitating the Working Alliance," the authors focus on the interpersonal skills that can be cultivated to promote a productive working alliance between therapist and client/patient. Specifically,

they identify pan-theoretical, pragmatic methods of improving therapist interpersonal skills with the goal of establishing and maintaining working alliances.
The authors then review the eight Facilitative Interpersonal Skills (FIS) and discuss the role of therapist responsiveness—the ability to detect and modify in-
session processes based on subtle, interpersonal shifts in the client's expression
and communication. Therapist responsiveness and the use of FIS is of particular
importance during challenging, emotionally charged incidents during therapy,
known as "critical relational markers." Finally, they discuss how therapists can
foster these relational capacities through deliberate practice. Clinical examples
are utilized to facilitate understanding of the application of these skills.

Chapter 4 is entitled "Setting Goals and Tasks in the Working Alliance" and
aims to facilitate the development of positive working alliances by providing
practitioners with the skills to set and develop attainable therapy goals and
methods to achieve goal consensus. These goals should be determined in collaboration with the patients, should be in the patients' best interest, and should
address the patients' problems. Once the therapist–patient dyad has established
the goals of therapy, they will need to collaborate on establishing the treatment
tasks that will help the patients achieve their goals. Finally, progress toward goals
should be assessed, and termination should be discussed from a goal perspective.
Moreover, therapists should discuss plans for the future with their patients, including an invitation to return to treatment if the need arises, as well as possible
referrals for additional help if necessary. The authors present clinical examples of
how to develop goals and tasks in therapy. Chapter 5 is entitled "Consensus and
Collaboration in the Working Alliance," and in it the authors address consensus
and collaboration, two related concepts that the authors believe are key to developing a positive working alliance. They discuss how to establish consensus and
collaboration with patients, as well as how consensus and collaboration evolve
from the beginning of treatment to termination. Additionally, they provide clinical examples of how to achieve consensus and collaboration within the working
alliance, and they discuss three interrelated markers of client behavior that signal
that there is consensus and collaboration in the client–therapist dyad: collaborative motivation, framework motivation, and collaborative action. The goal of this
chapter is to provide therapists with the tools to foster a "confident collaborative
relationship."

Chapter 6 is entitled "Clients' Perspectives on, Experiences of, and
Contributions to the Working Alliance: Implications for Clinicians" and focuses
on the other side (argued here as the more important side) of the working alliance: the clients' perspectives, experiences, and contributions. The authors
of this chapter provide a practice-friendly review of the research on the
clients' understandings of the alliance and offer suggestions and techniques
that professionals can use to develop and maintain a working alliance that is

responsive to clients' subjective understandings. Moreover, Chapter 6 aims to remind clinicians that the client's experience of the alliance is more predictive of successful counseling and psychotherapy than their own and that they should dedicate significant effort to the development of a working alliance that fosters openness and positive emotions. Particular emphasis should be placed on the early interactions in and prior to psychological treatment, the relational experience of interventions, and the value of micro-skills (i.e., validation) when developing and maintaining a working alliance. Chapter 7 is entitled "Multicultural Considerations in the Working Alliance" and addresses the importance of the working alliance from a multicultural perspective. To best serve the needs of racial/ethnic minority clients, it is critical to acknowledge and consider their differential social and cultural realities, as well as the therapists' own sociocultural contexts. Therapists may need to be intentional in their attempts to connect with racial/ethnic minority clients by developing appreciation and respect for cultural diversity. The appreciation and respect for cultural diversity that is developed from a therapist's self-work can then facilitate an open, accepting, honest, and empathic working relationship with racial/ethnic minority clients. The author of this chapter provides clinical examples and specific therapeutic skills that can foster the working alliance with racial/ethnic minority clients.

Chapter 8 is entitled "A Therapist's Guide to Repairing Ruptures in the Working Alliance," and in it the authors discuss the phenomena of "misattunements," or ruptures, in the working alliance. They present a set of skills and tools that aim to help therapists recognize and identify when ruptures occur, and they introduce a model for managing these moments. Albeit difficult, ruptures in the working alliance are common, and research shows that a therapist's ability to recognize and attend to these ruptures has a positive relationship with client improvement at the end of therapy. Strategies that have been successful in rupture repair (the therapist's attempts to address the rupture and restore the alliance with the client) include the therapist's exploration of the client's experience of the rupture and the acknowledgment of the client's perspective. Finally, they present real-world, clinical examples of their *stage-process model of rupture resolution*, which consists of strategies that can help therapists negotiate difficult therapeutic moments by employing the technique of mindfulness and demonstrating genuineness and authenticity in the therapist–client relationship. Chapter 9 is entitled "Facilitating Supervisee Competence in Developing and Maintaining Working Alliances: Supervisor Roles and Strategies" and focuses on the supervisor–supervisee relationship and its effect on the supervisee–client alliance. As detailed by the authors, the working relationship between a supervisor and a supervisee is paramount in the supervisee's professional development. The supervisor–supervisee relationship provides the contextual framework from which supervisees begin to form therapeutic alliances with their own clients.

In this chapter, the authors discuss the areas of supervisory focus that can improve the supervisee–client working alliance by focusing on specific attitudinal and skill-related issues that affect alliance-related competence. Finally, in Chapter 10, I discuss the most salient content in each of these chapters with the goal of highlighting themes and integrating ideas for the reader. I also discuss implications for future thinking with respect to training and clinical practice from the perspective of the working alliance.

We (and "we" includes all the authors in the book) certainly hope that you find these chapters helpful as a guide in thinking about what to do—and not do—in developing the working alliance. If you are a student in training, keep in mind that reading these chapters alone will not be enough. You must rely on your teachers, supervisors, and/or trusted colleagues for help and support in developing your own unique approach to working alliance development. If you are a professional in clinical practice, you may also benefit from reading some of the related literature on the psychotherapy relationship and from participating in continuing education activities available through state and national professional organizations. These activities will help you to enhance and complete your knowledge, competence, and skills in developing and sustaining strong and fruitful working alliances with your clients/patients.

References

American Psychological Association. (2012). Recognition of psychotherapy effectiveness. Retrieved from https://www.apa.org/about/policy/resolution-psychotherapy.aspx.

American Psychological Association, Commission on Accreditation. (2015). Standards of Accreditation for Health Service Psychology. Retrieved from http://www.apa.org/ed/accreditation/about/policies/standards-of-accreditation.pdf.

Bordin, E. S. (1979). The generalizability of the psychoanalytic concept of the working alliance. *Psychotherapy: Theory, Research & Practice, 16*(3), 252–260. http://dx.doi.org/10.1037/h0085885.

Castonguay, L. G., Constantino, M. J., & Holtforth, M. G. (2006). The working alliance: Where are we and where should we go?. *Psychotherapy: Theory, Research, Practice, Training, 43*(3), 271.

Constantino, M. J., Morrison, N. R., Coyne, A. E., & Howard, T. (2017). Exploring therapeutic alliance training in clinical and counseling psychology graduate programs. *Training and Education in Professional Psychology, 11*(4), 219–226.

Flückiger, C., Del Re, A. C., Wampold, B. E., & Horvath, A. O. (2018). The alliance in adult psychotherapy: A meta-analytic synthesis. *Psychotherapy, 55,* 316–340.

Freud, S. (1912/1990). The dynamics of transference. In R. Lang (Ed.), *Classics in psychoanalytic technique* (pp. 312–322). New York: Rowman & Littlefield.

Fuertes, J. N., Gelso, C. J., Owen, J. J., & Cheng, D. (2015). Using the Inventory of Countertransference Behavior as an observer-rated measure. *Psychoanalytic Psychotherapy, 29*(1), 38–56.

Gelso, C. J. (2002). Real relationship: The "something more" of psychotherapy. *Journal of Contemporary Psychotherapy, 32,* 35–41.

Gelso, C. J. (2011). *The real relationship in psychotherapy: The hidden foundation of change.* Washington, DC: American Psychological Association.

Gelso, C. J., & Carter, J. A. (1985). The relationship in counseling and psychotherapy: Components, consequences, and theoretical antecedents. *The Counseling Psychologist, 13*(2), 155–243. http://dx.doi.org/10.1177/0011000085132001.

Gelso, C. J., & Carter, J. A. (1994). Components of the psychotherapy relationship: Their interaction and unfolding during treatment. *Journal of Counseling* Psychology, *41*(3), 296–306. http://dx.doi.org/10.1037/0022-0167.41.3.296.

Gelso, C. J., Kivlighan Jr, D. M., & Markin, R. D. (2018). The real relationship and its role in psychotherapy outcome: A meta-analysis. *Psychotherapy, 55*(4), 434.

Greenson, R. R. (1967). The working alliance and the transference neurosis. *The Psychoanalytic Quarterly, 34*(2), 155–181.

Hayes, J. A., Gelso, C. J., Goldberg, S., & Kivlighan, D. M. (2018). Countertransference management and effective psychotherapy: Meta-analytic findings. *Psychotherapy, 55*(4), 496.

Horvath, A. O. (2001). The alliance. *Psychotherapy: Theory, Research, Practice, Training, 38*(4), 365–372. http://dx.doi.org/10.1037/0033-3204.38.4.365.

Horvath, A., & Bedi, R. (2002). The alliance. In J. C. Norcross (Ed.), *Psychotherapy relationships that work: Therapist contributions and responsiveness to patients* (pp. 37–69). New York, NY: Oxford University Press.

Horvath, A. O., Del Re, A. C., Flückiger, C., & Symonds, D. (2011). Alliance in individual psychotherapy. *Psychotherapy, 48*(1), 9.

Lambert, M. J., & Barley, D. E. (2001). Research summary on the therapeutic relationship and psychotherapy outcome. *Psychotherapy: Theory, research, practice, training, 38*(4), 357.

Levendosky, A. A., & Hopwood, C. J. (2016). A clinical science approach to training first year clinicians to navigate therapeutic relationships. *Journal of Psychotherapy Integration.* Advance online publication. http://dx.doi.org/10.1037/int0000042.

Sterba, R. (1940). The dynamics of the dissolution of the transference resistance. *Psychoanalytic Quarterly, 9,* 363–379.

Zetzel, E. R. (1956). Current concept of transference. *International Journal of Psychoanalysis, 37,* 369–376.

2

The Bond of the Working Alliance

Andrés E. Pérez-Rojas, Jazmin M. González, and Jairo N. Fuertes

The working alliance is that part of the overall therapy relationship that pertains to the working or professional connection between client and therapist (Gelso, 2014). As Fuertes noted in the Introduction to this volume, the working alliance has been defined as *the alignment or joining together of the client's reasonable self or ego with the therapist's analyzing or therapizing self or ego for the purpose of accomplishing the work of therapy* (Gelso & Carter, 1994). Said differently, the alliance is a collaborative process whereby client and therapist come together to observe, understand, and address the client's concerns.

For this collaborative process to unfold successfully, Bordin (1979, 1994) theorized that client and therapist must agree on the goals and tasks of therapy and form an emotional bond to support their shared activity. Thus, the bond of the alliance is best thought of as a *working bond*, an attachment that reflects the dyad's feelings and attitudes toward one another and that are rooted in their collaboration, allowing the work of therapy to get done (Hatcher & Barends, 2006). As such, the working bond differs from the primarily cognitive aspects of the alliance that emphasize consensus or negotiation about the goals of therapy and the tasks needed to achieve them (Horvath & Greenberg, 1989; Mallinckrodt & Tekie, 2016). It also differs from other types of bonds or interpersonal relationships between two or more people in that, as part of the alliance, this bond exists solely for the purpose of advancing the work of therapy.

The working bond, measured alongside the goals/tasks aspects of the alliance, is crucial to the process and outcome of therapy (see Flückiger, Del Re, Wampold, & Horvath, 2018). For this reason, it is important that therapists attend to it closely. In this chapter, we discuss what therapists can do to form, sustain, and end this bond successfully. First, we discuss the defining features of the bond per Bordin's (1979, 1994) tripartite model of the working alliance and briefly consider the demands that each of three major theoretical orientations (psychodynamic, humanistic-experiential, and cognitive-behavioral) place on this bond.

Next, we discuss what therapists can do, in general, to foster the working bond. Here, we briefly review the therapist-offered conditions that are core elements of

As in all chapters, the clinical material in this chapter is an amalgamation of clinical experiences. No one client can be identified.

Rogers's (1957) statement of the necessary and sufficient conditions for effective personality change. In our clinical experience, although therapists vary in their use of skills and the theoretical lens through which they view clients and their work, these facilitative conditions are robust ingredients of the working bond across theories and thus provide a useful framework for how to foster it.

Finally, we consider how the working bond unfolds throughout the stages of therapy in order to highlight factors which, in our experience, are important to attend to when building, maintaining, and terminating the bond. Throughout this section, we provide case examples from the literature and our own clinical experiences to illustrate salient processes.

Before proceeding, we should note that this chapter, in line with the rest of this volume, is geared toward practicing clinicians, especially those early in training. For those seeking a discussion of the working bond (and/or the working alliance as a whole) from a more empirical perspective, we suggest consulting Norcross (2011). We should also note that although the working bond is, naturally, a product of both the client and the therapist, our primary focus is on what the therapist can do during treatment to build and strengthen the bond.

Defining Features of the Working Bond

As we stated before, the working bond is that aspect of the working alliance that pertains to the more emotional experience and connection between client and therapist that supports the therapeutic work. What does this bond look like specifically, or how does it manifest in therapy? Bordin (1994) stated that the working bond "is likely to be expressed and felt in terms of liking, trusting, respect for each other, and a sense of common commitment and shared understanding" in the activities of therapy (p. 16). Thus, on a basic level, the bond involves feelings of trust, liking, and respect between client and therapist (see also Hatcher & Barends, 2006). Without trust, in particular, it is hard to imagine clients feeling safe or motivated enough to engage in any task common to all forms of therapy (e.g., sharing feelings) or those of specific treatments (e.g., systematic desensitization in cognitive-behavioral therapies). It is also difficult to envision a successful therapy that lacks mutual respect enabling client and therapist to approach one another effectively. Thus, the bond is evident when the client feels some connection to the therapist as a trusted, competent, and respected professional.

The bond is also said to have *work-potentiating qualities*—it instills a sense of confidence that the client–therapist collaboration will result in positive outcomes (Hatcher & Barends, 2006). In this sense, the bond manifests as the dyad's engagement and optimism for the treatment. The bond is also reflected in the client's confidence that the therapist can and sincerely wishes to help them, is on their side, and has their best interest at heart. Finally, a strong working bond is also manifest in the therapist's abiding commitment to help the client and their confidence in and appreciation for the client's efforts and capacity to heal.

There has been some debate in the literature as to whether some feelings, most notably *liking*, rightfully pertain to the working bond or to another component of the total therapy relationship: the *real relationship* (Bordin, 1994; Gelso, 2011). Recall from Fuertes's Introduction to this volume that the real relationship denotes the person-to-person relationship (as opposed to the working relationship, i.e., the working alliance) between client and therapist and that it is characterized by mutual genuineness as well as mutual perceptions that are realistic, accurate, or that befit who client and therapist really are (Gelso, 2011). This person-to-person relationship is particularly overlapping with the bond part of the working alliance (Gelso, 2014, p. 126). So when clients feel liking for their therapists, to what extent does that reflect their working bond (i.e., their professional connection)? And to what extent does it reflect their real relationship (i.e., the more person-to-person connection that forms whenever two people meet)?

Given this substantial overlap, it may seem like hair-splitting to try to distinguish whether clients like their therapists personally or professionally. Despite the overlap, however, many studies do indicate that the real relationship and the working bond contribute independently to the prediction of treatment progress and outcome (Gelso, 2014). In addition, recent evidence (Kivlighan, Kline, Gelso, & Hill, 2017) suggests that the real relationship and the working bond— measured alongside the goals/tasks dimension of the alliance—have similar *as well as* differential effects on how helpful and effective some clients find a therapy session, depending on whether the real relationship and the alliance are equal in strength or one is stronger than the other in a given session and throughout the therapy. These findings suggest that therapists need to attend closely to which aspect of the therapy relationship (i.e., the working bond as part of the alliance vs. the real relationship) is more salient or needed by each client and within each session. For that, it helps to consider these concepts' similarities and differences.

In all, although feelings of liking may undergird both a real relationship and a working bond, this does not diminish the importance for therapists to distinguish between these components when conceptualizing the therapeutic relationship in their work. For our purposes, a useful principle to keep in mind is that the core of the working bond is "joint purposive work" (Hatcher & Barends, 2006, p. 296). Said differently, the bond exists to support the goals and tasks of therapy (Bordin 1979, 1994), and, as such, it is a working bond, unlike other types of bonds (e.g., a friendship, a real relationship, etc.) or the relationship one may establish with other types of socially sanctioned healers (e.g., pastors, curanderos, tribal leaders, etc., although there are similarities between therapy and other socially sanctioned methods of healing; see Frank & Frank, 1991). The following case vignette serves to illustrates these points.

Dewayne sought therapy for depression following a difficult breakup. During therapy, Dewayne and his therapist worked together to better understand the internal narrative behind Dewayne's views of himself and how it fostered his depression. Dewayne appreciated his therapist and felt close to him as a trusted professional. The therapist, in turn, had positive feelings toward Dewayne as well. Their working bond was thus strong; the sense of trust, liking, and respect between them allowed them to work well together to help Dewayne heal. After some time, during which Dewayne gained much insight and was consistently depression-free, he and the therapist mutually agreed to end the treatment, thus ending their working bond, too. Dewayne would continue to feel appreciative of his therapist and the help he provided even after the treatment ended. He could even sometimes hear his therapist's voice in his head, which offered some comfort and even encouragement whenever he faced challenges in his life. But Dewayne neither wished nor needed to go back and speak with the actual therapist. Likewise, the therapist no longer wished or needed to see Dewayne. He still had positive feelings when thinking of Dewayne, but those feelings would not be described as a working bond, as there was no longer therapy work that needed to be supported with this therapy-related bond.

Thus, when thinking of the working bond, therapists may want to ask themselves some of these questions. How are they and their clients feeling about their working relationship? Do clients feel a sense of confidence in the therapist's skills? Do they feel like the therapist is emotionally invested in, supportive, and even optimistic about the therapy? Is there a sense of mutual caring and respect for one another as people engaged in collaborative work? To what degree is there a sense of partnership, collaboration, or shared mission in the relationship? These questions, by no means exhaustive, point to the distinctive features of the working bond.

The Working Bond Across Different Therapies

Bordin (1979, 1994) also proposed that different therapies place different demands on the bond of the alliance. Hence, what the alliance (and, within it, the working bond) may look like in practice may differ depending on the orientation of the treatment and the demands of the work. What sort of demands does each theoretical orientation place on clients and the working bond? To examine this question, we consider three major theoretical clusters that have had a great impact on the field: psychodynamic, humanistic-experiential, and cognitive-behavioral.

In the psychodynamic tradition, clients are asked to focus on the unconscious meanings and motivations behind their thoughts, feelings, and behaviors and their likely roots in early childhood (Gelso, Nutt Williams, & Fretz, 2014). To support this exploration and advance the work, psychodynamic therapists will likely focus on the client's transference toward the therapist (and the therapist's own countertransference) (Gelso et al., 2014). For some therapists, the working through of the transference is the central task of therapy; for others, transference interpretations serve mostly to illuminate client dynamics and foster insight. In either case, clients learn about themselves by exploring their interactions in the therapy relationship in some fashion (Murdock, 2017). Such intra- and inter-personal exploration can be quite threatening, emotionally, for clients, so it is easy to see why a strong working bond may be required. The working bond in these therapies can also facilitate the process of free association, the expression of repressed material, and the client's response to the therapist's interpretations. As Bordin (1979) noted, "when attention is directed toward the more protected recesses of inner experience, deeper bonds of trust and attachment are required and developed" (p. 254).

In the humanistic-experiential tradition, a premium is placed on clients' capacity to make their own rational decisions, actualize their full potential, and realize their own worth and dignity as human beings (Gelso et al., 2014). To support these aims, therapists under this theoretical umbrella engage in slightly different tasks that place certain demands on clients for which a strong working bond is helpful. For example, person-centered therapies require that clients abide by the nonactive/nondirective style of the therapist, who focuses on providing a climate of care, concern, and interest that will allow clients to unlock their own potential (Murdock, 2017). This might be rather difficult for clients who crave more guidance and structure to meet their goals. Other therapies under this cluster (e.g., gestalt, emotion-focused, etc.) are much more active/directive and place heavier emphasis on helping clients deepen and integrate their inner experiences within the here-and-now of the therapeutic relationship (Gelso et al., 2014; Murdock, 2017). This type of intervention may be quite challenging for some clients, too, as they may be unaccustomed to interacting with others in this rather intimate manner—and thus a strong foundation of trust and respect within the working bond is needed.

Finally, in the cognitive-behavioral tradition, the working bond is predicated on clients adopting more of a student-like role in order to learn new, helpful ways of thinking and behaving (Gelso et al., 2014; Murdock, 2017). At the same time, the client is also expected to serve as a collaborator "whose direct input is always solicited in setting session agendas and selecting home- work assignments" (Murdock, 2017, p. 325). The traditional cognitive- behavioral therapist will thus attend to the bond of the alliance to the extent that it can support the application of techniques and encourage clients to re- main engaged in activities or homework that build on what they are learning during sessions to modify their thinking and/or behavior. In contrast, a sound bond as part of the alliance appears to be more relevant in cognitive- behavioral treatments that are relatively less focused on specific techniques and interventions (e.g., mindfulness-based cognitive therapy; Jazaieri, Goldin, & Gross, 2018).

In sum, the major theoretical orientations place different demands on clients. The degree of trust, liking, respect, and collaboration required to successfully engage in those treatments will vary accordingly (Bordin, 1994; Hatcher & Barends, 2006). However, we must add that, despite this variation, all approaches do seem to require a degree of bonding that fosters trust and collaboration in the therapeutic work (Flückiger et al., 2018).

Facilitative Conditions: A Framework for Building and Sustaining the Working Bond

We have so far discussed defining qualities of the working bond: trust, liking, respect, and a sense of willing collaboration. We have also discussed how the kind of therapy and the demands placed on clients may affect this bond. Now we turn to how therapists may foster the defining features of the working bond to build and sustain it. We focus on a set of relational or facilitative conditions that contributes to making collaborative, purposeful work possible. In particular, we focus on the most widely known therapist-facilitating conditions—empathy, unconditional positive regard, and genuineness—which have roots in Rogers's (1957) statement of the necessary and sufficient conditions for effective thera- peutic change.

Perhaps one of the most audacious propositions in the history of psycho- therapy was Carl Rogers's (1957) suggestion that six conditions were necessary and sufficient, of themselves, to create effective client change in therapies of all orientations. These conditions are (a) the client and therapist are in psycholog- ical contact; (b) the client is in a state of incongruence, feeling anxious or vul- nerable; (c) the therapist is genuine or congruent in the relationship; (d) the therapist experiences unconditional positive regard for the client; (e) the ther- apist experiences an empathic understanding of the client's viewpoint and attempts to convey this to the client; and (f) the client perceives the therapist's empathy, positive regard, and congruence, at least to some extent.

Of the six conditions, those that pertain to the therapist (empathy, positive regard, and genuineness) have received the most attention since Rogers's (1957) formulation. A great deal of research over the years has indeed supported the importance of these therapist-offered conditions. However, although these conditions have been found to be therapeutic under most circumstances, they are not fully sufficient, as Rogers first suggested (Elliot, Bohart, Watson, & Greenberg, 2011; Farber & Doolin, 2011; Kolden, Klein, Wang, & Austin, 2011). What this means is that other factors are also involved in successful psychotherapy (e.g., techniques, other aspects of the therapy relationship, etc.; see Hill, 2014; Norcross, 2011). Still, decades of research have indeed established that the therapist's empathy, unconditional positive regard, and genuineness do seem to facilitate positive change in clients—particularly when assessed from the client's vantage point (Elliot et al., 2011; Farber & Doolin, 2011; Kolden et al., 2011).

Experiencing and conveying attitudes of empathy, positive regard, and genuineness are essential to engaging clients in a way that fosters the working bond. *Empathy*, in particular, allows therapists to partially identify with clients' inner worlds. This involves understanding clients from their frame of reference, tracking their emotional responses, validating their experiences, and evoking and clarifying underlying thoughts and feelings (Elliott et al., 2011). Using empathy, therapists can glean information that is essential to deciding what actions may be best to form and sustain the working bond depending on the client's unique needs and treatment goals (Hatcher, 2015). Being empathic can also help therapists deepen their clients' experiences and their capacity to reflect on their goals, feelings, and situations, further enabling the development of trust and of the working bond.

For its part, *unconditional positive regard* involves therapists' warm, enduring, and unqualified acceptance of clients (Farber & Doolin, 2011). Responding to clients in this manner frees them to say and experience anything in therapy without fear of judgment. Thus, clients are able to express what they need to, even if it is difficult or shameful, in order to achieve their treatment goals. Regarding clients positively and unconditionally also tells them that they matter to therapists—that they are liked and respected for who they are, fundamentally. As such, these features of positive regard (caring, liking, respect, etc.) are key ingredients in the working bond.

Finally, *genuineness* refers to therapists being open, self-aware, and authentic with clients (Kolden et al., 2011). This condition highlights the importance of therapists being aware and open to any aspect of their inner experience—both positive and negative—that may impact their ability to respond appropriately and provide a viable working bond to clients (Gelso & Perez-Rojas, 2017).

Moreover, if clients perceive that therapists are true to themselves in the therapeutic encounter, they may be more comfortable engaging collaboratively with them than if they perceive them as hiding behind a professional façade. Finally, sharing one's genuine self with clients, directly or indirectly, may model the type of honest disclosure that can enhance the working bond and the treatment (Kolden et al., 2011). This does not imply that therapists simply say whatever passes through their minds, only that they remain open to and aware of their thoughts and feelings and, if appropriate, share them with clients.

The therapist-offered conditions are often viewed as a set of relational skills that facilitate the therapist's use of more theory-specific techniques (e.g., Hatcher, 2015). Importantly, however, the conditions also reflect inner experiences or attitudes of valuing, accepting, and understanding clients that inform what therapists do in session (see Gelso & Perez-Rojas, 2017, for a discussion of the facilitative conditions as inner experiences). Used responsively to foster the working bond, these conditions set the stage for therapists to provide a climate of trust, liking, respect, and collaboration in the treatment. Indeed, being perceived as warm, empathic, and genuine has been found to influence the extent to which clients perceive therapists as trustworthy and credible (Hilsenroth, Cromer, & Ackerman, 2012). How therapists convey these attitudes to clients may be done in many ways. It may be done subtly, via eye contact, facial expression, and posture (Egan, 2010). Alternatively, it may be done more directly, via verbal cues or therapists' interventions that are consistent with their theoretical approach. The point is that virtually every skill or intervention can express a facilitative attitude. Those that convey warmth, active listening, empathic connection, and an authentic interest in the client's concerns and inner being have been found to predict the strength of the alliance (Hilsenroth et al., 2012) and are thus likely to foster the working bond.

The Working Bond in the Initial Phase of Psychotherapy

Having discussed the value for therapists to experience and convey attitudes of empathy, positive regard, and genuineness to foster the working bond, we now turn to how therapists may translate these attitudes into practice at different phases of psychotherapy, beginning with the initial phase. This phase, when client and therapist first come together and work toward initiating the treatment, is understandably a critical time for developing the working bond, as Gelso and Carter (1994) argued. The quality of the early bond (as measured by the degree of closeness, mutual engagement, and intimacy between client and therapy in the first two sessions), contributes greatly to the strength of the overall alliance in later sessions (Sexton, Littauer, Sexton, & Tømmerås, 2005). An early viable alliance, in turn, is a robust predictor of treatment success across differing approaches and treatment lengths (Flückiger et al., 2018). Hence, it is key to establish a bond of trust and cooperation with clients as early as possible.

In addition to the facilitative conditions, literature suggests that several therapist actions and qualities, not tied to any one theoretical orientation, positively affect the alliance early in treatment. According to Hilsenroth et al. (2012), it is important to attend to elements of the therapeutic frame, such as adopting a collaborative stance and doing involved, depth-oriented interviews, early on. The literature also suggests that the early alliance may be helped by allowing clients to initiate discussion of meaningful concerns, actively exploring those concerns, identifying recurrent themes in clients' issues, and focusing on and facilitating clients' emotions. Finally, therapists should foster some initial insight into clients' concerns, collaborate in developing treatment goals and tasks, and encourage motivation for change.

This literature does not distinguish whether such therapist actions and qualities influence the working bond more than, less than, or equally to the other parts of the alliance (agreement on goals and tasks). Yet, in our clinical experience, such attributes do affect the extent to which mutual trust and collaboration is developed and so they have a high likelihood of fostering the working bond, specifically, early in the work. In the next two sections, we focus on two factors, in particular, that we believe therapists must attend to at this early stage to build a sound working bond: the process of goal consensus and the client's capacity to trust.

Attending to the Bond in the Goal Consensus Process

During the initial phase of therapy, the earliest entry point to building a positive working bond may be the process of goal consensus. This process involves reaching agreement about the nature of the problem for which clients are seeking therapy, what they wish to get out of therapy, and what they will do with their therapist to achieve their goals (see Chapter 4 for more on setting goals and tasks). In this way, goal consensus represents an early marker of the ability of client and therapist to collaborate.

In addition, through the process of goal consensus, therapists glean valuable information about the type of working bond that clients may prefer, need, or find helpful. A classic qualitative study (Bachelor, 1995) helps to illustrate what we mean. In this study, Bachelor asked a sample of 34 counseling center clients what they viewed as a good client–therapist working relationship at various points in therapy (including during the initial stage). The responses clustered into three groups: 46% of clients stressed the importance of therapists being respectful, nonjudgmental, empathic, and attentive (labeled a "nurturant alliance"); 39% stressed therapists' actions that provide clarification and insight (labeled an "insight-oriented alliance"); and 16% stressed more of a sense of mutuality, or a recognition that the therapeutic process involves contributions from both the client and the therapist (labeled a "collaborative alliance"). Importantly, for nearly all clients in the Bachelor (1995) study, facilitative conditions similar to the Rogerian conditions were considered very consequential, irrespective of the type of alliance into which the clients clustered. Many subsequent findings have been largely consistent with those of Bachelor's study (see review by Hilsenroth et al., 2012).

Although by no means set in stone, Bachelor's (1995) results serve as useful illustrations or templates with which to think about the type of working bonds that could support a client's goals and sustain the tasks of therapy (Hatcher & Barends, 2006). Do clients want or need therapists to foster a bond that is consistent with a nurturant, insight-oriented, or collaborative alliance, as identified by Bachelor? Or do they need another type of working bond altogether—one that was not captured in that study? One should also consider the sorts of tasks clients are willing to engage in to make changes and how they fit into the therapist's theoretical orientation. As we discussed earlier, Bordin (1979, 1994) theorized that different types of therapeutic tasks (and thus different therapies) place different demands on the working bond. Thus, it is wise to tailor the bond to the tasks of the particular type of treatment to which the client has agreed and entered. This is consistent with Egan's (2010) notion of establishing what he called a *just society*, a relationship "based on mutual respect and planning. Therefore, establish as much mutuality as is consonant with helping goals" (p. 123).

As we noted, Bachelor (1995) also found that most clients still valued qualities reflecting the therapist-offered conditions, irrespective of the type of alliance they preferred. As such, therapists should not neglect these conditions when determining the type of working bond to build, regardless of their theoretical preferences. To show genuine interest and care in the consensus process, for example, therapists may pair questions about clients' concerns and goals with gentle, follow-up probes. Probes also encourage depth of exploration, which is positively related to the strength of the early alliance (Hilsenroth et al., 2012). The early alliance is stronger when therapists attend to in-session affect, speak in emotional and cognitive terms, affirm and support clients, remain focused on clients' concerns, and do not provide too much advice or information (Hilsenroth et al., 2012). Some ways of enacting these behaviors include reflecting feelings (e.g., "You sound hopeful"), restating (e.g., "You have doubts about your relationship"), validating (e.g., "How frustrating that must have felt"), and using evocative language (e.g., "It's like you're thrashing about in a net; you feel trapped, helpless") (Elliot et al., 2011; Hill, 2014).

The following case vignette illustrates how to apply the preceding principles to attend to the working bond in the process of goal consensus.

THERAPIST: Thank you for being so open, James. We have covered a lot of ground today, and I'm curious if you have a sense of what feels like a priority for us to focus on?

JAMES: Hmm. I don't know. Everything seems important! I guess. . . . Maybe if I could just meet someone, get married, have kids, make more money, I'll be happier! You think you can give me all that? [Chuckles nervously.]

THERAPIST: [Smiling] If I could do all that, I think I'd be a magician or something, or at least I'd be a much richer therapist, you know? [Therapist shows an authentic, humorous side of her personality and makes a small joke to help ease James's nervousness.]

JAMES: [Less nervous] Ha-ha, that's true.

THERAPIST: In all seriousness, realistically, I can't promise you'll find someone and be happily married after doing therapy. What we can do, though, is put our heads together and explore what's been getting in the way of relationships for you. How does that sound? [Therapist adopts a collaborative stance to address James's concerns.]

JAMES: Yeah, I guess that sounds okay. [Pauses. Looks down.]

THERAPIST: I notice you looked away, James. Can you share with me how you're feeling? [Therapist is unsure, but senses an important feeling was triggered and moves to explore.]

JAMES: I mean, what you said is good. But I just wonder, is it worth it? Like, maybe there's something wrong with me. Why can't I just figure this out? Everyone else seems to know how to meet people and talk to them and. . . . Ugh. I don't even know where to start figuring out something like this, something that seems so basic to everyone else.

THERAPIST: [Trying to meet James' gaze kindly.] You sound almost overwhelmed, James. I can really hear it in your voice. I don't think there's anything wrong with you. This is actually really hard stuff—painful, even. And I really respect you for having the courage to seek therapy to try to do something about it. [Therapist empathically reflects salient affect in James's expression and conveys positive regard, disclosing her own perception that there is nothing wrong with James and providing initial support and reassurance.]

JAMES: [Meeting her gaze] Yeah. Thank you.

THERAPIST: You're welcome. And, you know, I'm actually hopeful that together we can figure out a way for you to feel better and for things to be different. [Therapist conveys hope for the treatment and uses language that stresses collaboration and togetherness.]

JAMES: [Seeming relieved.] You really think so?

THERAPIST: I do. We don't have to figure it all out right this second; we can take our time. But you won't be doing it alone.

JAMES: That sounds good. And it actually does feel a little better to talk about this with someone, for once.

THERAPIST: That sounds great. And so different from what you said just a moment ago, doesn't it? When you said you didn't know where to even start figuring this out. Do you notice a difference? How are you feeling right now? [Therapist calls attention to the difference in James's affect.]

JAMES: Better. [Pauses.] I don't know, sometimes I feel really down about it, you know? I guess I always thought that everything in my life would feel more settled right now.

THERAPIST: "More settled." Hmm. That sounds really important. Help me understand what "most settled" feels like for you. [Therapist focuses in on affect and fosters depth.]

In this example, the therapist invited James to identify treatment goals and tasks as part of the process of goal consensus. Sensing James's unease, however, she shifted to focusing more explicitly on their working bond. Embodying the facilitative conditions, the therapist targeted core features of this bond: trust, liking, respect, collaboration, and confidence in the treatment's potential to alleviate distress (Bordin, 1979, 1994; Hatcher & Barends, 2006). Indeed, through a calming and accepting attitude and the use of exploratory reflections and restatements, the therapist conveyed concern and attention to James's issues and his experience in therapy, which helped to build her credibility and fostered their budding connection.

After this intervention, the work may follow a number of different directions, depending on James's eventual goals and the therapist's theoretical leanings. A psychodynamic therapist, for example, might focus on the unconscious associations James has to the notion of a "more settled life," while a cognitive-behavioral therapist might unpack the core beliefs at the root of James's thought process. No matter what theory-specific tasks James and his therapist eventually engage in, the preceding approach is well aligned with literature on therapist actions and attributes that are associated with viable early working alliances across theories (Hilsenroth et al., 2012) and thus are likely to have a positive effect on the working bond itself.

In the vignette, the therapist responded to James's need for care and support rather than the need to nail down specific treatment goals right away. Judging by James's response and his willingness to disclose more vulnerable feelings, he seemed to appreciate the approach. In this way, he may have indicated a preference for a more nurturant-type of bond and alliance, one that involves building a sense of ease, trust, and support to promote more disclosure (Bachelor, 1995). Of course, rather than surmise clients' preferences in this manner, therapists may well ask what they are looking for from the therapist. This may be done via immediacy (Hill & Knox, 2009) or by engaging clients in a role induction or psychoeducation process, which involves orienting clients to salient aspects of the treatment and assessing expectations (Swift & Greenberg, 2015). In our experience, clarifying both parties' expectations about their roles in therapy can normalize how clients experience the working bond and the therapeutic relationship as a whole—which is, after all, a unique type of relationship. The discussion may also delineate what both client and therapist would find acceptable in their interactions, thereby anchoring their working bond in the principle of a "just society" (Egan, 2010).

Attending to the Client's Capacity to Trust

An important factor that therapists should attend to when developing the working bond is the client's capacity to trust (Gelso et al., 2014). It is not surprising that trust is vital to forming the bond, as we have argued, since trust is vital to forming healthy and secure relationships in general. How trust develops over time, in turn, is influenced by people's attachment patterns, which have to do with how comfortable people are being close with others and how secure they feel depending on and having others depend on them (see Mikulincer & Shaver, 2007). This applies to therapy, as well: studies show that clients' attachment patterns are related to their ability to eventually trust their therapists, feel secure in therapy, and contribute to the development of the therapeutic relationship (Strauss & Petrowski, 2017; Wiseman, 2017).

Hence, therapists may wish to inquire about the quality of their clients' bonds, especially earlier in life, as these early interactions shape later attachment experiences, including their ability to sustain trust and intimacy. Of course, therapists should also consider their own early experiences, attachment patterns, capacity for trust and intimacy, and the degree to which these will affect their ability to foster and sustain a sound bond. Ultimately, the goal should be to actively meet clients where they are, as it were, with respect to their capacity to participate meaningfully in a close, intimate, and trusting therapy relationship from the start of treatment to its eventual conclusion (see Wiseman, 2017, for further discussion of these points). Assuming that clients will automatically trust their therapists—without making at least some effort to meet them where they are—is counterproductive to the development of a working bond.

The client's capacity to trust others must also be understood within the context of culture. Clients' cultural values and worldviews may impact the extent to which they feel it is permissible to rely on others outside of their communities or their families, including therapists, for help (Asnaani & Hofmann, 2012). For members of cultural minority groups, there may also be a degree of justifiable cultural mistrust toward medical and mental health professionals due to prior institutional exploitation and oppression (APA Multicultural Guidelines; American Psychological Association [APA], 2017). For these and various other reasons, it is important that therapists explore and address cultural factors that may impinge on clients' capacity to trust others and have a positive experience in therapy (see Chapter 7 for more on multicultural issues in the working alliance).

The following example illustrates how to attend and respond with warmth, empathy, and genuineness to early signs that a client may not feel fully trusting in therapy.

Julia is a 22-year-old, cisgender, straight woman of Afro-Caribbean descent. She seeks therapy due to depressive symptoms that have persisted for more than 3 months. This exchange takes place during the second session of therapy.

JULIA: I'd say I get along with my parents. But lately it's been kind of tense or hard? [Pauses. Seems nervous.] I don't know. I've been pretty down these last few months, like I've been saying. And my parents can tell something's up with me. But I don't want to bother them with. . . . [Pauses. Wrings hands.] Yeah, they have enough to . . . worry about.

THERAPIST: You seem nervous, Julia. [Therapist reflects Julia's feelings to draw attention to her in-the-moment experience.]

JULIA: Yeah, I don't know. [Silence.]

THERAPIST: It seems like it's harder for you to talk about this than anything else we've talked about so far. I'm wondering, is there something about our relationship, or being in therapy, that might be contributing to that? [Sensing Julia's apprehension, the therapist attempts to explore potential mistrust of the therapist or the therapeutic process.]

JULIA: Well, now that you mention it, it's kind of awkward bringing this up. I don't know, this is family business. And in my family we always keep our problems to ourselves.

THERAPIST: Yeah, you keep it in the family. So how is it telling me—someone who's not in your family—about this? [Therapist uses immediacy to home in on Julia's misgivings about discussing family matters with the therapist, specifically.]

JULIA: It's hard. Like, don't get me wrong, I think you're very nice and you've been pretty helpful already. And I'm so glad I'm finally in therapy because, like I said last week, I'm so sick of feeling down like, all the time. But it's hard. It's awkward. We just tend to keep things in the family, where I'm from.

THERAPIST: I'm glad to hear this has felt helpful so far, Julia. But I also hear this can be hard, too. It seems like part of you feels uncomfortable talking about family.

JULIA: Yeah.

THERAPIST: And I'm wondering if part of you also feels like you'd be disrespecting or betraying their cultural values by talking about it with me? What do you think? [Therapist reflects Julia's feelings and reassures her. Picking up on her statement "where I'm from," the therapist asks whether Julia's cultural values contribute to her reservations.]

JULIA: Oh wow. I hadn't thought about it like that, but yeah. My culture's part of it, too. [Pauses. Becomes teary.] That's hard, too, you know? In my culture, we like to say that our lives are not just our own to live. As my parents' child, I'm supposed to live for them, do everything I can to honor and make them happy. And it hurts to think that maybe I'm not doing that. That I'm disappointing them somehow.

THERAPIST: That sounds really painful, Julia. And really important. There's a part of me that really wants to hear more about how you feel, and what your culture and family mean to you. But I'm aware that talking about these things might feel uncomfortable. So maybe we can first talk about what's okay and not okay to talk about outside your family? That might make it a little easier for you. [Therapist discloses his authentic "pull" toward exploring Julia's feelings but instead takes the opportunity to process how he and Julia could establish a bond that honors her cultural values.]

In this vignette, we illustrate how therapists can intervene when encountering distrust or apprehension on the client's part. Here, the therapist's empathic ability helps him grasp that, in this cultural context, Julia is being asked to flout family values grounded in her ethnic culture. Consistent with the principles of positive regard and establishing a "just society" (Egan, 2010), the therapist prompts an open dialogue about how to explore relevant family and cultural dynamics in a way that fits and feels comfortable for Julia. The therapist's actions also embody *cultural humility*, which involves being open, curious, respectful, nonassuming, and authentic when attending to salient aspects of clients' cultural identities (Davis et al., 2018). As can be seen, the qualities of a culturally humble approach overlap greatly with the Rogerian facilitative conditions. After their conversation, Julia seemed more open and trusting in therapy, secure in the knowledge that the therapist was responsive to her needs and cultural values. The conversation also helped the therapist later in treatment to use certain interventions (e.g., interpretations of early family dynamics) in a similarly responsive manner.

The Working Bond in the Working Phase of Psychotherapy

Once client and therapist have formed a sound working bond and reached an understanding of how to collaborate in therapy, they move to what may be termed a *working phase*. This phase looks different depending on the therapist's orientation, case conceptualization, treatment strategies, and the theory-specific tasks that client and therapist engage in to achieve treatment goals. In general, however, the aim here is for client and therapist to engage together in the often-arduous work of helping the client change.

How does the working bond unfold during this phase? In many ways, the working bond can be expected to deepen. As the work intensifies and clients feel better and begin to make changes, they may become more hopeful and feel closer to the therapist (Larsen & Stege, 2012; Luborsky, 1976). Therapists, in turn, foster closeness by using techniques that are supportive (e.g., affirm client's experiences), exploratory (e.g., clarify areas of distress), experiential (e.g., explore different emotions), and engaging (e.g., focus on the here-and-now of the therapeutic relationship) to convey understanding, connectedness, collaboration, and to enhance clients' own understanding of their concerns (Hilsenroth et al., 2012). Since these techniques help advance clients' goals, it makes sense that this would foster the working bond (Hatcher & Barends, 2006).

In many cases, however, the working bond does not follow a strictly linear or stable path as the work deepens. In fact, there is evidence that the bond (measured alongside goals/tasks) can follow certain high-low-high trajectories that are actually linked to more favorable outcomes than are stable or linear trajectories (Horvath, Del Re, Flückiger, & Symonds, 2011). The findings are mixed, however, and the literature does not have definitive answers for why these patterns occur, why they are linked to more positive outcomes, or how best to respond to them.

In our experience, these fluctuations in the bond and the alliance speak to the rigors of the working phase of psychotherapy. This is the time when clients are doing the heaviest lifting, psychologically speaking. They are seeing things differently; they are learning new ways of thinking, feeling, and behaving; and they are adjusting to changes that are often scary or painful to make. All of this can certainly put strains on clients and the bond, affecting its strength. Bordin (1994) himself alluded to such strains in the alliance, a concept which has now been extended and heavily studied by others over the years (e.g., Safran & Muran, 2000). In particular, some authors have argued that fluctuations in the working bond may correspond to periods in therapy when there are ruptures in the alliance, which may be thought of as more severe forms of alliance strains. Alliance ruptures, when repaired, can enhance the treatment. When left unaddressed, however, they can impede the on-going client–therapist collaboration and harm the work.

Given these possible trajectories and their potential effects on the outcome of therapy, therapists would do well to track and assess the quality of the bond as treatment progresses and attend to any ruptures that occur along the way. Here, we expand on these points and provide relevant case examples. We should note that our discussion of alliance ruptures will be brief, and more extensive cov-erage of this topic will be given elsewhere in this volume (Chapter 8).

Assessing the Strength of the Working Bond

How can therapists monitor the strength of the bond in the working phase (and beyond)? One way is to attend closely to fluctuations in one's own feelings, mining them for clues about what may be happening in the relationship. Recognizing and attending to one's feelings is, of course, an important aspect of the Rogerian con-dition of genuineness, as explained before. Using their self-awareness, therapists may reflect on how they feel about the working relationship. Have they noticed differences compared to when the work started? Do they still like and respect the client as someone engaged in the arduous work of therapy? We recognize that sometimes these questions may be uncomfortable, especially when therapists have negative reactions to clients, and more so if these reactions are tied to areas of vulnerability or unresolved conflicts in the therapist (i.e., countertransference; Gelso & Hayes, 2007). It is normal, however, to experience a range of reactions to clients—positive, negative, and countertransference-based. Allowing oneself to know, accept, and experience these reactions is an important part of managing them to benefit the treatment (Gelso & Perez-Rojas, 2017), which includes using them to monitor the quality of the working bond as therapy progresses.

An awareness and understanding of one's experience of the working bond are important, but so, too, is attending to the client's experience of the bond. After all, evidence suggests that clients' perceptions of the working alliance are dif-ferent (see Chapter 6) and are often better predictors of treatment outcomes (cf. Flückiger et al., 2018). Therapists may focus on the defining markers of the working bond, as we discussed earlier in the chapter. Do clients continue to feel a sense of trust, respect, and collaboration? Do they seem to feel safe and under-stood? Are they confident in the therapist's ability to help them? And are these qualities present to a degree that allows "full endorsement of the goals and full participation in the tasks?" (Hatcher & Barends, 2006, p. 293). Therapists may go further and directly ask clients for their feedback about the working relationship. For example, they might say:

THERAPIST: You've been working very hard, Amina, these last few sessions. I wanted to take a moment and ask, how are you feeling about the way we're working together?

Although this type of intervention is often associated with more experiential treatments, virtually every theory sees direct communication about the working bond (and the therapeutic relationship more broadly) as a way to assess how clients are experiencing the bond and to address problems in the relationship (Hill & Knox, 2009). Beyond pointing out potential areas of remediation, directly communicating about the bond can enhance it by making clients feel accepted and understood, for example, and by providing a model for how to communicate openly in relationships outside of therapy—provided that such direct communication is relevant to the treatment and the client can tolerate such a style of interaction (Hill & Knox, 2009).

Another way to elicit client feedback is to use standardized session-to-session measures of treatment progress. A great deal of research has shown benefits to using client monitoring systems that provide feedback to therapists on clients' progress and experiences of the therapeutic relationship, regardless of therapeutic approach (Lambert & Shimokawa, 2011). An apt example is the Partners for Change Outcome Management System (PCOMS), which provides a brief session-by-session assessment of clients' reports of the alliance and treatment outcomes (Duncan & Reese, 2015). Research shows that using such client feedback reduces dropout rates, and further benefits are seen when the feedback is discussed with clients in session (Reese, Norsworthy, & Rowlands, 2009). The following example illustrates this approach.

Mateo and his therapist had been working for seven sessions. The agency where the work takes place asks clients to complete a measure that tracks their perceptions of treatment outcomes, as well as the goals, tasks, and bond dimensions of the working alliance, on a routine basis. The measure is scored electronically and the results are given to the therapist for inspection. Before today's session, the therapist notices that Mateo's alliance scores have been trending lower than in previous sessions.

THERAPIST: Before we start, I wanted to go over the results of the survey you've been taking here. As always, thank you for this feedback; it's incredibly useful. So, if I am reading this correctly, it looks like you left our last session feeling less heard, understood, and/or respected than other times. This is important to me, so could we talk about this?

MATEO: Well, last time we were talking about my anxiety and you told me about those mindfulness techniques to calm down. Those were helpful, but I don't know, I was really wanting us to also talk about my thoughts and my feelings, like we'd been doing before. But you kept focusing just on the mindfulness.

THERAPIST: Oh, I see. Thank you for sharing this with me, Mateo. Looking back, I can see how caught up I got in making sure you had tools to cope with the anxiety and I really didn't do a good job of hearing or understanding you. I'm sorry about that. [Therapist validates Mateo's perception, self-discloses his own experiences to help Mateo understand what happened, and apologizes.]

MATEO: Yeah, it's okay. I mean, I do think the mindfulness stuff can help, and I tried it a little and it kind of worked.

THERAPIST: Right, it sounds like those techniques can help, but it's important to me that you continue to feel heard and understood, even as we try different things to help you manage your anxiety. Maybe we can talk a little bit more about this?

Here, the therapist relied on an electronic system to track client feedback. Systems like the PCOMS and many other psychometrically sound feedback measures are available for free and take only a few minutes to administer and score, either manually or via widely used programs such as Excel (Duncan & Reese, 2015). Regardless of what format is used, what is important is to monitor the quality of the bond systematically and to use the results as a stepping stone to a discussion with the client. The discussion must be done warmly, empathically, collaboratively, and in a way that fits the therapist's style—otherwise clients may not feel safe enough to voice their honest views about the relationship. But, even without the use of formal monitoring systems, therapists would do well to periodically inquire about the health of their bonds with clients.

Repairing Ruptures in the Working Bond

As the preceding section shows, sometimes therapists miss things as they engage clients more intensely in therapy. Asking for feedback, as we argued, can fill in those blind spots and ensure that clients continue to feel connected to the therapist and to the work. Acting on that feedback, however, is the essential step that can help restore the strength of the bond if and when it falls below earlier, higher levels. For that, a framework of alliance rupture-repair may be useful.

What are alliance ruptures? Safran, Muran, and Eubanks-Carter (2011) defined them as "a tension or breakdown in the collaborative relationship between patient and therapist" (p. 224). These ruptures may be caused partly by a client's problematic interpersonal patterns (which are reenacted in therapy) and partly by interruptions in the therapist's empathic ability, both of which can cause frictions within the alliance. Ruptures may be unnerving for both client and therapist, but they provide opportunities to work with clients to understand and repair the ruptures, which ultimately can move the therapy forward (Safran et al., 2011).

In our experience, ruptures may occur on any aspect of the alliance. A rupture in goals and/or tasks, for instance, may indicate that client and therapist no longer agree on the nature of their work and what they are trying to achieve together. To repair this type of rupture, the therapist may ask the client if they can revisit their agreed-upon goals or to review the therapeutic activities they have engaged in to that point. In such cases, the working bond may remain relatively intact. Ruptures to the working bond itself, on the other hand, imply a breakdown in the sense of mutual trust, liking, and respect underlying the collaboration.

How might therapists go about repairing ruptures to the relational bond of the alliance? In general, the literature (e.g., Hilsenroth et al., 2012; Safran & Muran, 2000; Safran et al., 2011) suggests that once such a rupture is recognized, therapists invite clients to process it. Here, therapists use exploratory skills, empathic reflections, and subjective feedback about the rupture to support clients' communication. Therapists should also own their contribution to the rupture and further empower clients to express their feelings about the therapist directly. Finally, therapists adopt an affirming, accepting, and nurturing stance as they facilitate an understanding of the rupture, explore the meaning behind clients' feelings and experience of the rupture, and note similarities to past and present relationship difficulties. There is evidence that many therapists follow these strategies; however, therapists-in-training may struggle in particular with conceptualizing their role in the rupture and making connections between what happened with the therapist and the clients' relationships outside of therapy (Kline et al., 2018).

The following case (adapted from Kline et al., 2018) illustrates the process of repairing a rupture in the working bond.

The client (a 28-year-old woman) and the therapist-in-training had worked together for six sessions at a community clinic. The client had recently run a race and enthusiastically shared her results with the therapist. The therapist, eager to focus on the client's concerns instead, asked only cursory questions about the race before changing the subject. The client became upset. She said the therapist did not appreciate how important the race was to her and that her previous therapist would have understood. The client left the session feeling hurt and unappreciated. The therapist, in turn, felt shaken and overcome with anxious thoughts.

With her supervisor's help, the therapist reflected on her actions and came to understand how they connected to her fears of not being or doing enough to help her clients. Supervision provided a safe space to work through these feelings, reframe her anxious thoughts, and role-play ways to reconnect with the client. It also helped the therapist to reground herself in the facilitative attitudes and the spirit of collaboration that characterizes the alliance.

In the next session, the therapist asked the client if they could go back to what had happened between them in the last session. She apologized and acknowledged that how she reacted to the client's accomplishment was minimizing and, indeed, not how her previous therapist would have reacted. She further invited the client to share her feelings with the therapist directly. At times it was necessary to affirm and explore the client's fears about expressing negative feelings about the therapist. Throughout the discussion, the therapist asked open-ended questions to explore and arrive at a better understanding of the rupture and what the therapist should do differently in the future. The therapist also related what happened in the session with the client's experience outside of therapy and the themes they had been exploring in the work prior to the rupture. Although she felt nervous during this discussion, the therapist remained present, nonjudgmental, and empathically attuned to the client.

Afterward, the client said she felt more trusting of and understood by the therapist, partly because recognizing her mistake signified to the client that the therapist really respected her. Also, the therapist making an effort to explore her experience of the rupture and how it related to the client's concerns signified that she was committed to helping the client achieve her goals. All of this made the client feel more capable of being open than even before the rupture happened, which furthered the therapeutic work. The therapist still felt some lingering anxiety, but she was more confident in her ability to notice and repair potential ruptures.

We hope that the knowledge that strains or ruptures in the bond (and the other aspects of the alliance; see Chapter 8) can be repaired, and that doing so can facilitate the therapy process, is comforting to therapists—especially beginning clinicians who, in our experience, sometimes hold back from engaging more deeply with clients for fear that they will do or say something that damages the relationship. Holding back may "protect" the bond (or the self of the therapist) from the understandable discomfort that accompanies ruptures, but this can deprive clients of meaningful opportunities to change and achieve their goals. The mandate of the working bond and the alliance in general is, after all, to support therapeutic work. The guidelines discussed here and in other chapters may thus help therapists to use the bonds that they build with their clients to work with ruptures therapeutically when needed.

The Working Bond in the Termination Phase of Psychotherapy

The termination phase of psychotherapy is the period during which client and therapist consciously or unconsciously work toward ending the therapy (Gelso & Woodhouse, 2002). It differs from premature termination or client dropout, which occurs when clients end therapy unilaterally, before achieving goals or recovering from the concerns for which they sought help (Swift & Greenberg, 2015). Such cases may indicate that a viable alliance never actually developed or took hold or that ruptures in either the goals/tasks or the bond of the alliance went unrepaired. Whatever the case, premature terminations typically occur without much warning. Successful termination, in turn, is often planned, although this will vary depending on the circumstances of the termination. Whether client, therapist, or both initiate it because they feel the client has achieved their goals, or whether it is prompted by agency restrictions on treatment length or other outside factors, a successful termination process is an opportunity for client and therapist to work together to effectively end the treatment (Gelso & Woodhouse, 2002).

An important part of what makes termination effective is the therapist's attention to the working bond. Indeed, studies on clients' and therapists' views during termination reveal that the extent to which this phase is seen as positive depends, in great part, on the strength of the alliance (Bhatia & Gelso, 2017; Knox et al., 2011). A strong alliance (which includes a strong working bond) during termination, as rated by therapists, is also a significant predictor of overall treatment success, in contrast to other components of the relationship (i.e., transference and real relationship; Bhatia & Gelso, 2017). This evidence is ambiguous, however, in that the studies focus on the global alliance and do not break down results according to the goals/tasks and bond dimensions. Still, it makes clinical sense that the strength of the working bond, specifically, would facilitate this phase of treatment. For instance, the working bond may provide a great deal of support and stability during a process which, for some clients and therapists—especially those with a history of painful losses—may be rather difficult (Gelso & Woodhouse, 2002). For most, however, termination actually represents a time of pride, excitement, and consolidation (Quintana, 1993)—a reflection that clients have achieved their goals and, perhaps, that the bond contributed greatly to that process. Finally, how therapists attend to the working bond during termination may determine whether clients return to therapy if needed, either with the same therapist or with a different clinician. Thus, in many ways, the better the bond, the better the end.

Some therapists, mostly those who adhere to psychodynamic and humanistic-experiential orientations, tend to prescribe an explicit focus on the bond and other aspects of the relationship during termination (Curtis, 2002; Greenberg, 2002), whereas cognitive-behavioral therapists tend to advocate for focusing less on the relationship and more on maintaining gains (Goldfried, 2002). What most therapists do in practice, however, seems to actually involve both foci. Norcross, Zimmerman, Greenberg, and Swift (2017) recently queried a panel of expert therapists from diverse orientations about the frequency with which they engage in certain tasks during termination. There was far more consensus than disagreement in their responses. Some responses involved tasks for which a strong working bond would seem to be necessary (e.g., encouraging clients to maintain changes without the therapist's aid). Other termination tasks, in turn, implicitly or explicitly seemed to call for attending to the working bond itself (and other components of the therapeutic relationship) as the treatment draws to a close (e.g., processing feelings about ending the relationship and acknowledging the collaborative bond).

Our own clinically based impression is that, indeed, the working bond both affects and is affected by what transpires in the termination phase. The manner in which the treatment ends and what client and therapist do to end it tend to reflect the degree of mutual trust, liking, and respect present at that point in therapy. And the quality of the bond, in turn, greatly shapes the extent to which client and therapist can openly reflect on the journey they have undertaken and where the client needs to go once they part ways. Hence, it is important for therapists to set the stage for talking about termination. One method for doing so, which we explicate and illustrate here, involves helping the client to *look back* on what was worked on, *look forward* to the client's future, and *say goodbye* (Gelso & Woodhouse, 2002).

Looking Back

In looking back, client and therapist review the issues that have been discussed in therapy and the extent to which goals have been accomplished. Therapists assist clients in reflecting how they have changed or grown and, as needed, allow clients to voice what they liked and disliked about the treatment. The process of looking back still requires the therapist to engage clients with the warmth, empathy, and genuineness they strived to experience and convey throughout the treatment. And, in the spirit of the working alliance, the process should be done collaboratively, as well, with both client and therapist sharing their respective views of what they did together and what happened during their working relationship. For example, therapists may help clients to recognize and own the gains they made by pointing out clients' continued engagement in the treatment. Therapists may also encourage clients to share their feelings about the therapist directly and, in turn, share their own feelings regarding what it was like to work with the client. Goode, Park, Parkin, Tompkins, and Swift (2017) even suggested that therapists share their feelings about any mistakes they made during the course of therapy.

A case vignette presented by Goode et al. (2017) helps to illustrate the process of looking back during termination.

THERAPIST: It sounds like you feel like the gains you experienced over the last 18 sessions came from your willingness to start to explore your feelings, and thoughts, and regrets all surrounding your wife's death. It was difficult, but I am sure glad that you did it.

CLIENT: Yeah . . . I am, too. And I am grateful that you were here to help me do it. You gave me the encouragement to think about these things, and you seemed like you were able to put things together in a way that I was not able to do on my own.

THERAPIST: Well, I am glad I got to be part of this. It was neat to see you process some of the feelings that you had been avoiding. And, from my perspective, although I was there to help guide at times, you were really the one that brought it all together. [Pause.] You know, in life it seems like relationships always have their ups and downs. Although things went pretty smoothly while we worked together, I feel like there were a couple times when maybe I made mistakes, too. I remember back around the sixth or seventh session when we were talking about some of the regrets you had when your wife died, and I suggested that part of you was glad not to have the burden of the relationship any more. I was really off with that, and I am glad that you pointed it out to me.

CLIENT: Yeah . . . I was pretty mad. I thought about never coming back.

THERAPIST: I could see how mad you were, and I do appreciate the second chance. I am glad that even though I was not a perfect therapist, we were able to keep trying, and in the end it worked out pretty well. (pp. 12–13).

In this exchange, client and therapist are able to look back, review gains, and even share their mutual feelings about a rupture that took place in their bond. In this way, the process of looking back reinforces that both client and therapist have valuable insights into the work and that both collaborated to make the experience what it was. Some questions we have found helpful to ask ourselves or even pose to clients directly when looking back include: What has the client learned? How have they changed or grown? What were some turning points during the treatment? What is the client proudest of? What does the client wish the therapist would have done differently? And what did and did not work for the client?

Looking Forward

In looking forward, client and therapist discuss what issues remain to be resolved and the client's plans and hopes for the future. The discussion is, again, done collaboratively in an effort to jointly develop a plan for the client's continued growth (Goode et al., 2017). Planning for the future may include a conversation about what clients can expect once treatment ends, what resources exist for continued support, and how to anticipate and respond to relapse. It also includes discussion of whether it is possible to return to the same therapist for more treatment, if and when the client feels the need for further therapy, or if appropriate referrals need to be made.

The following case example helps to illustrate this aspect of termination.

Client and therapist have just reviewed the progress the client made in therapy.

THERAPIST: So you have a lot of new tools and a better understanding of yourself. Now, we did quite a bit of work in these 12 sessions, but I know there's more you wish we had time to work on. Can we talk about that? What feels unfinished for you?

CLIENT: Well, I want to see how things go with my partner now that I understand my feelings better, especially when we get into arguments. And I want to keep trying to be open with her, because even the little bit I have been doing has been really helpful. But I do notice that I still get a little scared about sharing how I feel, so I can see that being something I need to keep working on.

THERAPIST: That's a really good observation. You definitely made a lot of strides in that area but I hear you want to keep working on sharing your feelings. So, what exactly do you mean by that? And how do you see yourself being able to continue working on it?

CLIENT: It'd be nice if I wasn't afraid at all! But I know now that's not really realistic, and it's better if I can work on tolerating my fears. I think it'll help to remember that. And to remind myself that it's okay for me to ask for what I want and need. That's been a really good thing to realize and to practice doing.

THERAPIST: Yeah, that's really powerful. And that's something I've seen you do more of even in here, with me. So I'm confident that you can continue doing it.

CLIENT: Yeah, talking about things with you has definitely helped with that. It's been a little scary at times, for sure, but it's also made me feel more confident that I can do it with other people, especially my partner. So thank you.

This vignette highlights that even in cases where clients make tremendous progress, there may remain unresolved issues. Therapists thus serve their clients well by acknowledging and facilitating an open discussion about this and the client's vision for their future, regardless of whether the client and the therapist mutually establish a final date or termination occurs because of outside constraints. Also, consistent with the literature on termination (Gelso & Woodhouse, 2002), in looking forward the therapist may invite the client back for further treatment, if needed, which can help remind the client that they retain the therapist's support and, in this way, consolidate their memory of a positive working bond.

Saying Goodbye

Once client and therapist have looked back and looked ahead to the client's future, they are ready to say goodbye. Client and therapist can bring some closure to their relationship by focusing on what it has meant and what it feels like now that their relationship and the treatment are ending (Gelso & Woodhouse, 2002). It is important to devote as much time as necessary to explore and process what it means for clients to say goodbye. After all, for some, building a bond such as the working bond is in itself an important therapeutic outcome, and it is possible these clients may not have had healthy experiences around goodbyes or ending such bonds in everyday life.

Thus, therapists may wish to ask clients whether ending the working bond is similar (or not) to other important relationship endings. Moreover, do clients have a history of significant losses which may be triggered or revisited during termination (Gelso & Woodhouse, 2002)? Or do they experience more bittersweet feelings—a mixture of pride for ending treatment successfully and sadness about saying goodbye to the therapist? Often we have asked clients to share what comes to mind when they think about *saying goodbye* and how they typically do it, in an effort to explore and incorporate their cultural and personal beliefs and traditions around goodbyes. Throughout this process, it is important that therapists continue to communicate warmth and empathically affirm the client's experience of the termination.

Saying goodbye also involves the therapist sharing what the therapeutic relationship has meant for them and how they feel about the ending. Doing so aligns with the collaborative nature of the working bond that therapists strived to foster throughout the treatment and, as such, can consolidate the client's memory of therapy as a process characterized by trust and collaboration (Goode et al., 2017). Thus, as clients share their feelings about ending the bond, therapists should share their own feelings and experiences surrounding the bond, especially in a way that validates the client's contribution to the process. In many cases, more of the real relationship may emerge at this point as client and therapist relate to each other more as equals and the client can better see the therapist realistically (Curtis, 2002; Greenberg, 2002).

Another case example from Goode et al. (2017) serves to illustrate the reciprocal process of saying goodbye during a termination session.

THERAPIST: As we say goodbye, let me say that it has been an absolute privilege to go through this journey with you. It takes a lot of courage to open up to someone else, especially when the person is a stranger to you, and I appreciate you trusting me enough to share things that are very meaningful to you.

CLIENT: Well, it was easy to share with you. I didn't feel like you judged me, and that helped.

THERAPIST: I know you talked earlier about all the ways that you have grown over the course of therapy, but I wanted to make sure to acknowledge that this was a growing process for both of us. Because of these experiences interacting and learning with you, I feel I have grown as a therapist and as a person. You helped give me new ideas for how to help other people cope with stress in their lives, and, on a more important level, you taught me more about the resilience of people. So thank you. (p. 13)

For some clients, saying goodbye is more of a "see you later," as they may wish to return to the therapist in the future. Therapists should not take for granted, however, how a break of any length may influence the working bond. Also, in some cases, it may not be possible to return to the same therapist for treatment (e.g., when therapists-in-training leave an agency at the end of a rotation). For these and other reasons, as discussed previously, therapists should be prepared to process their own and their clients' feelings about ending the therapeutic relationship.

How much time to devote to saying goodbye (and to termination in general) will depend on many factors, like the therapist's theoretical orientation, the extent to which client concerns are resolved, and the length of therapy. Some studies suggest that 10–12% of therapy is typically devoted to termination (Gelso & Woodhouse, 2002). In our experience, there is great variability in this regard. We have even worked successfully with clients for several months, and all they seemed to need was a brief discussion to mark the end of therapy. Still, research does suggest that most clients want and need something akin to a termination phase (Gelso & Woodhouse, 2002). In our view, the model we just described may be conducted as formally or informally as therapists see fit or as needed by clients. The bottom line is that therapists should be thoughtful in how they approach ending the working bond with their clients during termination.

Summary

We have suggested that the working bond reflects the degree of mutual trust, liking, and respect that exists between client and therapist and that permits them to work collaboratively and withstand the demands of therapeutic work. Therapists can foster a sound working bond throughout treatment by experiencing and conveying the facilitative attitudes of empathy, positive regard, and genuineness. In the beginning, therapists should deploy these facilitative attitudes to build an early viable bond, paying close attention to the process of goal consensus and the client's capacity to trust others. During the working phase, therapists should closely monitor their own and their clients' sense of the working bond and attend to any ruptures that may threaten it. Finally, therapists may facilitate the successful termination of the working bond by engaging clients in a process of looking back over the work, looking forward to the client's future, and saying goodbye, all in a manner that preserves the spirit of warmth, acceptance, understanding, and collaboration that was present throughout the treatment.

References

American Psychological Association (APA). (2017). *Multicultural guidelines: An ecological approach to context, identity, and intersectionality.* Retrieved from http://www.apa.org/about/policy/multicultural-guidelines.pdf

Asnaani, A., & Hofmann, S. G. (2012). Collaboration in multicultural therapy: Establishing a strong therapeutic alliance across cultural lines. *Journal of Clinical Psychology, 68*(2), 187–197. doi:10.1002/jclp.21829

Bachelor, A. (1995). Clients' perception of the therapeutic alliance: A qualitative analysis. *Journal of Counseling Psychology, 42*(3), 323–337. doi:10.1037/0022-0167.42.3.323

Bhatia, A., & Gelso, C. J. (2017). The termination phase: Therapists' perspective on the therapeutic relationship and outcome. *Psychotherapy, 54*(1), 76–87. http://dx.doi.org/10.1037/pst0000100

Bordin, E. S. (1979). The generalizability of the psychoanalytic concept of the working alliance. *Psychotherapy: Theory, Research, and Practice, 16,* 252–260. http://dx.doi.org/10.1037/h0085885

Bordin, E. S. (1994). Theory and research on the therapeutic working alliance: New directions. In A. O. Horvath & L. S. Greenberg (Eds.), *The working alliance: Theory, research and practice* (pp. 13–37). New York: Wiley.

Curtis, R. (2002). Termination from a psychoanalytic perspective. *Journal of Psychotherapy Integration, 12,* 350–357. http://dx.doi.org/10.1037/1053-0479.12.3.350

Davis, D. E., DeBlaere, C., Owen, J., Hook, J. N., Rivera, D. P., Choe, E., . . . Placeres, V. (2018). The multicultural orientation framework: A narrative review. *Psychotherapy, 55*(1), 89–100. doi:10.1037/pst0000160

Duncan, B. L., & Reese, R. J. (2015). The Partners for Change Outcome Management System (PCOMS) revisiting the client's frame of reference. *Psychotherapy, 52*(4), 391–401. http://dx.doi.org/10.1037/pst0000026

Egan, G. (2010). *The skilled helper: A problem management and opportunity development approach to helping* (9th ed.). Pacific Grove, CA: Brooks/Cole Cengage Learning.

Elliott, R., Bohart, A. C., Watson, J. C., & Greenberg, L. S. (2011). Empathy. *Psychotherapy, 48*(1), 43–49. http://dx.doi.org/10.1037/a0022187

Farber, B. A., & Doolin, E. M. (2011). Positive regard. *Psychotherapy, 48*(1), 58–64. http://dx.doi.org/10.1037/a0022141

Frank, J. D., & Frank, J. B. (1991). *Persuasion and healing: A comparative study of psychotherapy* (3rd ed.). Baltimore, MD: Johns Hopkins University Press.

Flückiger, C., Del Re, A. C., Wampold, B. E., & Horvath, A. O. (2018). The alliance in adult psychotherapy: A meta-analytic synthesis. *Psychotherapy.* doi:10.1037/pst0000172

Gelso, C. (2014). A tripartite model of the therapeutic relationship: Theory, research, and practice. *Psychotherapy Research, 24*(2), 117–131. doi:10.1080/10503307.2013.845920

Gelso, C. J. (2011). *The real relationship in psychotherapy: The hidden foundation of change.* Washington, DC: American Psychological Association. doi:10.1037/12349-000

Gelso, C. J., & Carter, J. (1994). Components of the psychotherapy relationship: Their interaction and unfolding during treatment. *Journal of Counseling Psychology, 41*(3), 296–306. doi:10.1037/0022-0167.41.3.296.

Gelso, C. J., & Hayes, J. A. (2007). *Countertransference and the therapist's inner experience: Perils and possibilities.* Mahwah, NJ: Lawrence Erlbaum Associates Publishers.

Gelso, C. J., Nutt Williams, E., & Fretz, B. R. (2014). *Counseling psychology.* Washington, DC: American Psychological Association.

Gelso, C. J., & Perez-Rojas, A. E. (2017). Inner experience and the good therapist. In L. G. Castonguay & C. E. Hill (Eds.), *How and why are some therapists better than others?* (pp. 101–116). Washington, DC: American Psychological Association.

Gelso, C. J., & Woodhouse, S. S. (2002). The termination of psychotherapy: What research tells us about the process of ending treatment. In G. S. Tryon (Ed.), *Counseling based on process research: Applying what we know* (pp. 344–369). Boston, MA: Allyn & Bacon.

Goldfried, M. R. (2002). A cognitive-behavioral perspective on termination. *Journal of Psychotherapy Integration, 12,* 364–372. http://dx.doi.org/10.1037/1053-0479. 12.3.364

Goode, J., Park, J., Parkin, S., Tompkins, K. A., & Swift, J. K. (2017). A collaborative approach to psychotherapy termination. *Psychotherapy, 54*(1), 10–14. http://dx.doi.org/ 10.1037/pst0000085

Greenberg, L. S. (2002). Termination of experiential therapy. *Journal of Psychotherapy Integration, 12,* 358–363. http://dx.doi.org/10.1037/1053-0479.12.3.358.

Hatcher, R. L. (2015). Interpersonal competencies: Responsiveness, technique, and training in psychotherapy. *American Psychologist, 70*(8), 747–757. doi:10.1037/ a0039803

Hatcher, R. L., & Barends, A. W. (2006). How a return to theory could help alliance research. *Psychotherapy: Theory, Research, Practice, Training, 43*(3), 292–299. doi:10.1037/0033-3204.43.3.292

Hill, C. E. (2014). *Helping skills: Facilitating exploration, insight, and action* (4th ed.). Washington, DC: American Psychological Association.

Hill, C. E., & Knox, S. (2009). Processing the therapeutic relationship. *Psychotherapy Research, 19*(1), 13–29. doi:10.1080/10503300802621206

Hilsenroth M. J., Cromer T. D., & Ackerman S. J. (2012). How to make practical use of therapeutic alliance research in your clinical work. In R. Levy, J. Ablon, & H. Kächele (Eds.), *Psychodynamic psychotherapy research* (pp. 361–380). Totowa, NJ: Humana Press. https://doi.org/10.1007/978-1-60761-792-1

Horvath, A. O., Del Re, A. C., Flückiger, C., & Symonds, D. (2011). Alliance in individual psychotherapy. *Psychotherapy, 48*(1), 9–16. doi:10.1037/a0022186

Horvath, A. O., & Greenberg, L. S. (1989). Development and validation of the Working Alliance Inventory. *Journal of Counseling Psychology, 36,* 223–233. doi:10.1037/ 0022-0167.36.2.223

Jazaieri, H., Goldin, P. R., & Gross, J. J. (2018). The role of working alliance in CBT and MBSR for social anxiety disorder. *Mindfulness.* doi:10.1007/s12671-017-0877-9

Kivlighan, D. M., Jr., Kline, K., Gelso, C. J., & Hill, C. E. (2017). Congruence and discrepancy between working alliance and real relationship: Variance decomposition and response surface analyses. *Journal of Counseling Psychology, 64*(4), 394–409. doi:10.1037/ cou0000216

Kline, K. V., Hill, C. E., Morris, T., O'Connor, S., Sappington, R., Vernay, C., . . . Okuno, H. (2018). Ruptures in psychotherapy: Experiences of therapist trainees. *Psychotherapy Research.* doi:10.1080/10503307.2018.1492164

Knox, S., Adrians, N., Everson, E., Hess, S., Hill, C., & Crook-Lyon, R. (2011). Clients' perspectives on therapy termination. *Psychotherapy Research, 21*(2), 154–167. doi:10.1080/10503307.2010.534509

Kolden, G. G., Klein, M. H., Wang, C.-C., & Austin, S. B. (2011). Congruence/genuineness. *Psychotherapy, 48*(1), 65–71. http://dx.doi.org/10.1037/a0022064

Lambert, M. J., & Shimokawa, K. (2011). Collecting client feedback. In J. C. Norcross (Ed.), *Psychotherapy relationships that work: Evidence-based responsiveness* (2nd ed., pp. 203–223). New York: Oxford University Press. doi:10.1093/acprof:oso/9780199737208.003.0010

Larsen, D. J., & Stege, R. (2012). Client accounts of hope in early counseling sessions: A qualitative study. *Journal of Counseling & Development, 90*(1), 45–54. doi:10.1111/j.1556-6676.2012.00007.x

Luborsky, L. (1976). Helping alliance in psychotherapy. In J. L. Cleghhorn (Ed.), *Successful psychotherapy* (pp. 92–116). New York: Brunner/Mazel.

Mallinckrodt, B., & Tekie, Y. T. (2016). Item response theory analysis of Working Alliance Inventory, revised response format, and new Brief Alliance Inventory. *Psychotherapy Research, 26*(6), 694–718. doi:10.1080/10503307.2015.1061718

Mikulincer, M., & Shaver, P. R. (2007). *Attachment patterns in adulthood: Structure, dynamics and change.* New York: Guilford Press.

Safran, J. D., & Muran, J. C. (2000). *Negotiating the therapeutic alliance: A relational treatment guide.* New York, NY, US: Guilford Press.

Murdock, N. L. (2017). *Theories of counseling and psychotherapy: A case approach* (4th ed.). New York: Pearson.

Norcross, J. C. (Ed.) (2011). *Psychotherapy relationships that work: Therapist contributions and responsiveness to patients* (2nd ed.). New York: Oxford University Press.

Norcross, J. C., Zimmerman, B. E., Greenberg, R. P., & Swift, J. K. (2017). Do all therapists do that when saying goodbye? A study of commonalities in termination behaviors. *Psychotherapy, 54*(1), 66–75. http://dx.doi.org/10.1037/pst0000097

Quintana, S. M. (1993). Toward an expanded and updated conceptualization of termination: Implications for short-term, individual psychotherapy. *Professional Psychology: Research and Practice, 24,* 426–432. http://dx.doi.org/10.1037/0735-7028.24.4.426

Reese, R. J., Norsworthy, L. A., & Rowlands, S. R. (2009). Does a continuous feedback system improve psychotherapy outcome? *Psychotherapy: Theory, Research, Practice, Training, 46*(4), 418–431. http://dx.doi.org/10.1037/a0017901

Rogers, C. (1957). The necessary and sufficient conditions of therapeutic personality change. *Journal of Consulting Psychology, 21*(2), 95–103.

Safran, J. D., & Muran, J. C. (2000). *Negotiating the therapeutic alliance: A relational treatment guide.* New York: Guilford Press.

Safran, J. D., Muran, J. C., & Eubanks-Carter, C. (2011). Repairing alliance ruptures. In J. C. Norcross (Ed.), *Psychotherapy relationships that work* (2nd ed., pp. 224–238). New York: Oxford University Press.

Sexton, H., Littauer, H., Sexton, A., & Tømmerås, E. (2005). Building an alliance: Early therapy process and the client–therapist connection. *Psychotherapy Research, 15*(1-2), 103–116. https://doi.org/10.1080/10503300512331327083

Strauss, B. M., & Petrowski, K. (2017). The role of the therapist's attachment in the process and outcome of psychotherapy. In L. G. Castonguay, & C. E. Hill (Eds.), *How and why are some therapists better than others?* (pp. 139–158). Washington, DC: American Psychological Association.

Swift, J. K., & Greenberg, R. P. (2015). *Premature termination in psychotherapy: Strategies for engaging clients and improving outcomes.* Washington, DC: American Psychological Association. http://dx.doi.org/10.1037/14469-000

Wiseman, H. (2017). The quest for connection in interpersonal and therapeutic relationships. *Psychotherapy Research, 27*(4), 469–487. https://doi.org/10.1080/10503307.2015.1119327

3

Therapeutic Interpersonal Skills for Facilitating the Working Alliance

Timothy Anderson and Matthew R. Perlman

This chapter focuses on how therapists can identify and cultivate skills for building a positive and productive therapeutic alliance with their clients. Surprisingly, therapists and trainees have relatively few resources for learning the practical elements of alliance development. What skills can a therapist learn for building therapeutic relationships with clients? Qualitative data from clinical psychology training sites across the United States and Canada have found that, while most programs largely believe in the importance of the alliance, training sites largely had no systematic training curricula on helping new trainee therapists learn to develop an alliance with clients (Constantino, Morrison, Coyne, & Howard, 2017). Given this gap, our aim for this chapter will be to identify pragmatic methods for improving therapist interpersonal skills in forming and maintaining working alliances.

Most often, alliance-building skills have been addressed in the context of the traditional supervisory model of clinical training; however, building alliance-enhancing skills through traditional supervised therapy cases and accumulative clinical experience may not be the best route for improvement in alliance formation and maintenance. Accumulating therapeutic experience, without attending to the specific skills, may not lead to improvements in the therapeutic alliance or client outcomes (Wampold & Brown, 2005). An inordinate focus on following the specific techniques of a given treatment may actually distract therapists from attending to the interpersonal space between client and therapists. In fact, one study found evidence that those therapists who best adhere to treatment techniques were also more prone to undermine the therapeutic relationship (Henry et al., 1993) even while being highly responsive to utilizing supervision and the specific treatment techniques (Anderson et al., 2012). It is remarkable that these negative side effects were associated with a year-long training that was designed to enhance therapists' abilities to address the therapeutic relationship!

Recent focus has been given to training individual therapists to build the therapeutic alliance by building individual alliance skills, though there have been challenges. Smith-Hansen, Constantino, Piselli, and Remen (2011) developed and tested the effects of teaching therapists to enhance the therapeutic alliance through an alliance building workshop, and Crits-Christoph and colleagues (2006) developed a specific treatment manual for building the therapeutic alliance. While their innovative training attempts established that training was feasible, the outcomes were less encouraging, which may have been due to small samples and methodological limitations.

What might be done to enhance training therapists to build better alliance? Our approach for how therapists can improve their therapeutic alliances is premised on two important foundations. First, the skills that therapists learn to enhance therapeutic alliances should be common or pan-theoretical—after all, the therapeutic alliance is a pan-theoretical construct (Bordin, 1979), and it makes some sense that the skills that therapist learn to enhance the alliance also would be pan-theoretical or, at minimum, specific skills that can be flexibly adapted to multiple treatments. While on this topic, it's important to note that this does not imply that therapists should avoid specificity. As described by Hatcher and Barends (2006), the distinction between specific treatments and the alliance (or relationship) is something of a false dichotomy. The therapeutic alliance includes techniques, in the form of task agreement, but it is defined primarily by the sense of collaboration and genuine agreement on those tasks. Our point may seem somewhat esoteric, but it is important to stress that therapists' abilities to know specific treatments is an important contributor to good alliance; nonetheless, the skills for building the therapeutic alliance are more comprehensive, common, and contextual in nature. Second, the most promising avenues for building individual alliance skills are linked to what is known about which therapist skills and characteristics are most associated with good client outcomes.

Why Focus on Therapists?

Over the past decade, more research attention has been given to the critical effects of the therapist in psychotherapy process and outcomes. While some originally viewed therapist effects as a "nuisance" variable or a confound to be controlled for, more recent investigations have found that individual therapists demonstrate consistent differences that have robust impacts on treatment process and outcome. For example, Laska, Smith, Wislocki, Minami, and Wampold (2013) investigated the effect of 25 therapists who were delivering a uniform therapy protocol to a sample of 192 veterans in the treatment of posttraumatic stress disorder (PTSD). The results showed that an astounding 12% of the variance in outcome was accounted for by therapist effects.

Meta-analytic data show that therapists typically account for somewhere between 5% and 8% of the variance in client outcomes (Baldwin & Imel, 2013). As a point of comparison, meta-analytic data show that the type of treatment used (e.g., cognitive-behavioral therapy [CBT], psychodynamic, client-centered, etc.) accounts for less than 1% of the variability in clinical outcomes (Wampold et al., 1997). Most data do not support the idea that there is some type of interaction between therapists and treatment techniques driving these large therapist effects. Research instead shows that the differences among therapists goes above and beyond the specific techniques and treatments that they are using. Summarizing available research on the topic via a meta-analysis, Webb, DeRubeis, and Barber (2010) found that therapist adherence to techniques accounted for a mere 1% of their client's outcomes. Clearly, therapists have a demonstrable effect on the course of therapy via mechanisms other than the treatment being utilized.

What makes some therapists more effective than others may include some of the same factors that makes the working alliance the best process-level predictor of client outcomes. Thus, it would be extremely helpful to know which therapist skills are contributing to their better outcomes and how those skills can be used to bolster a stronger therapeutic alliance. Systematic research on therapist effects and skills has found that effective therapists tend to possess significantly greater *facilitative interpersonal skills* (FIS; Anderson, Ogles, & Weis, 1999, Anderson, Crowley, Himawan, Holmberg, & Uhlin, 2015; Anderson, McClintock, Himawan, Song, & Patterson, 2016) than do less effective therapists. Perhaps not surprisingly, high FIS therapists also had significantly higher working alliances, too (Anderson et al., 2015). Identifying more effective therapists allows us to shed a light on what effective, alliance-enhancing therapists may be doing during these critical markers. FIS operates on the premise that high-performing therapists distinguish themselves during the most challenging moments of sessions. Some clients move through therapy as highly engaged and collaborative to the point where almost any therapeutic task and goal, even the most questionable, would be approached positively. In these situations, therapists of any level of interpersonal ability would likely be able to foster a positive relationship and, ultimately, treatment outcome.

There is much utility in therapists' ability to respond to the most challenging interpersonal moments, those moments that have the greatest potential to damage the working alliance. Research on FIS has found that responses to such critical relational markers, albeit brief moments, carry considerable weight when it comes to good outcomes and the working alliance. While these common skills of FIS, in total, and their emergence within critical moments appear to be important, the therapist's abilities to adjust, adapt, and reflexively respond to the intensity of moments with clients are a more encompassing skill. This skill has been referred to as *responsiveness* (Stiles, Honos-Webb, & Surko, 1998), and it is unclear if responsiveness is the more broad-based and encompassing skill or if

FIS serves this role. Nonetheless, it is necessary to introduce the skill of therapist responsiveness at the same time as introducing the set of FIS.

Identifying Alliance Skills Through Responsiveness to Critical Relational Markers

As a well-identified general practice concept for building effective alliances and therapy outcomes, the therapist's *responsiveness* (Stiles et al., 1998) refers to the ability of a therapist to detect and modify in-session processes based on subtle, interpersonal shifts in the client's expression and communication. It's notable that therapist responsiveness is not a specific behavior or technique that a therapist can *explicitly* learn because it is integrally linked to both what the client expresses and what the client needs. Thus, therapists can only be responsive after they have gained a competent understanding of the client's experience (using interpersonal aptitudes such as empathy, which will be discussed later in the chapter). Instead of a skill/technique, responsiveness would better be conceptualized for our purposes as a relational *capacity*. We believe that practice and experience using the skills and concepts described in this chapter represent a strong foundation on which to build the capacity for responsiveness.

What may best distinguish therapists' interpersonal skills is their responsiveness to demanding, often emotionally charged, incidents during therapy. We call these incidents "critical relational markers." These markers may separate "the wheat from the chaff" of therapeutic skills for numerous reasons, one of which is that important moments are meaningful to clients while being extremely activating for therapist. This type of scenario can be considered a form of "performance under pressure." Critical relational markers can signal for the client whether their therapist is trustworthy, invested, and engaged in their relationship. Negative responses within those critical moments may also reveal reasons for the client to be distrustful of the therapist, negatively impacting both the working alliance and the overall process of therapy.

Facilitative Interpersonal Skills: Measuring Therapist Responsiveness

While therapist effects are a robust predictor of process/outcome, and qualities such as responsiveness offer us a framework for understanding complex interpersonal processes, we have not yet described a way to consider what, exactly, the best therapists do in their sessions to foster strong relationships. This is where the specific facets of the FIS paradigm come into play. Drawn from clinical observation, theory, and research (Anderson et al., 1999; Anderson & Strupp, 2015), the FIS are a set of eight key relational capacities which are robustly linked to therapy process and outcome. In a series of rigorous empirical investigations, Tim Anderson and colleagues have found that FIS predicts therapy outcome over and above self-reported social skills, age (i.e., years of experience), and demographic factors (Anderson et al., 2009). A second FIS investigation compared training status (i.e., advanced graduate students in clinical psychology vs. untrained students in non-helping profession such as chemistry or art history) to interpersonal abilities (i.e., FIS and social skills). The results showed that someone's FIS, *not* their level training as a therapist, predicted their alliance and outcomes with clients in therapy (Anderson et al., 2015). A final study revealed that FIS, assessed in clinical psychology graduate students in their first month of school, predicted client outcomes in therapies which were conducted *more than a year later* (Anderson et al., 2016). Ultimately, these results show that FIS are a robust, long-term indicator of therapist interpersonal capacities.

The eight skills of the FIS are assessed through the FIS task. The task is a computer-administered protocol where study participants respond to a series of professionally acted video stimulus clips which are all drawn from real therapy sessions. The stimulus clips represent various forms of critical relational markers, demonstrating a variety of interpersonal challenges. In some of these challenges, simulated clients have trouble opening up to the therapist. In other clips, the simulated clients may be overtly criticizing some aspects of the process of treatment.

The unique computer-based format allows the FIS task to see how participants respond to challenging, high-pressure clinical scenarios in a standardized way. Given the significant variability of real-world clients, the FIS task provides us with a way of equitably assessing the performance of different therapists as they respond to the exact same situations via the stimulus clips. Responses to clips are typically video and audio recorded. Then, a trained team codes and rates the clips on a 1 ("not characteristic") to 5 ("highly characteristic") scale for the eight FIS: verbal fluency, emotional expression, hope/positive expectations, persuasiveness, warmth/acceptance/understanding, empathy, alliance bond capacity, and alliance rupture repair responsiveness (ARRR).

FIS: Understanding the Eight Skills

Verbal fluency measures the comfort and smoothness of the participant's message. Highly verbally fluent responses sound relaxed, well-paced, and feature an almost rhythmic quality. Low verbal fluency is often indicated via expressions of anxiety in communicating: stammering, awkward/extended pauses, and a lack of clarity in speech. Verbal fluency is less about the content of the message and more focused on the vocal qualities or way the message is delivered.

Emotional expression, much like verbal fluency, focuses on the delivery of the response as opposed to its verbal content. The energy and feeling associated with the message's conveyance are ways of characterizing emotional expression. Highly emotionally expressive FIS responses are engaging, show clear affect, and have a strong prosody. Responses lacking emotional expression appear dull, flat, and feature little affect.

Hope/positive expectations reflects how optimistic or positive a message is. This is coded, primarily, through the content of the message. An FIS response high in hope/positive expectations will demonstrate a believable, personalized pathway for the simulated client to recover and make changes. The best responses also allude to the fostering of the client's agency in building these positive pathways. Responses low in hope/positive expectations will often show overt pessimism, describe the issue as out of the client's control, and have an air of hopelessness about them.

Persuasiveness corresponds to the capacity of a response to encourage and convince a client to accept a new perspective, understanding, or a way forward. Highly persuasive responses are personally tailored to fit the issue at hand, use clear/understandable language, and feel convincing. Messages low in persuasiveness feel generic, lack credibility, or may even be incoherent.

Warmth/acceptance/understanding is another FIS item that requires coders to detect the attitude or feeling of a message along with its content. Showing high warmth/acceptance/understanding refers to a therapist's ability to demonstrate genuine care for the client, to accept them as they are, and to show compassion even while trying to help the client change. Responses low in warmth/acceptance/understanding reveal a judgmental attitude, guilt-induction, and even exasperation or annoyance with the client. Some especially poor responses will overtly blame the client for their current position without demonstrating any understanding of the complex context that got them there.

Empathy refers to the level of understanding shown for the client's subjective experience. In other words, to what extent does the therapist understand, and attempt to show this understanding of, the client's perspective on the issue at hand? Highly empathic FIS responses show that the participant has clearly listened closely, uses the client's language, and even inferred some of the less explicit aspects of the client's experience. Responses low in empathy disregard the simulated client's experience, distort what the client has said or feels, and may clearly misidentify obvious aspects of the client's situation.

Alliance bond capacity shows how skilled a response is at fostering a collaborative atmosphere for tackling the critical relational marker. Responses demonstrating strong alliance bond capacity will ensure that the problem(s) is/are being worked on as a team, make active efforts to engage the client as part of the problem-solving process, and may even check in with the client to ensure that they have an accurate understanding of the situation that works for both parties. Responses lacking in alliance bond capacity will typically undermine the fostering of a collaboration by putting much (or all) of the responsibility on the simulated client or even moralistically lecturing the client on how to proceed.

Finally, *alliance rupture repair responsiveness* rates how attuned and receptive the participant is to the issue at hand. Each simulated client presents with a unique interpersonal issue (or "rupture") with their therapist which requires an individualized solution. Responses high in ARRR will not only detect this issue as it pertains to the immediate process between client and therapist, but they will also act on responding to these issues. Good ARRR can be seen through discussing what is occurring in the session, as opposed to trying to pivot to situations which may or may not be happening *outside* of therapy, and will attempt to incorporate both client *and* therapist perspectives in developing a resolution. Responses low in ARRR will typically miss the critical interpersonal marker entirely. When the marker is identified and acted on in a response demonstrating poor ARRR, it is done so in a way that deepens the issue. Most often, this is accomplished through hostility and taking control (both subtle and overt).

In research, FIS ratings are averaged together to get a composite score across the eight skills. At a conceptual level, the skills are interdependent. For example, to provide a targeted, persuasive message of hope, one should have a solid, empathic understanding of a client's inner world. To adequately repair a rupture, one must be able to form a collaborative bond. As such, we will present these skills in theoretically linked clusters as we discuss methods for training and enhancing skills.

Using FIS as a Basis for Clinical Training

Research on these therapeutic processes and therapist effects is highly suggestive that individual therapists likely differ in skills and individual characteristics that facilitate a strong therapeutic relationship (Anderson & Hill, 2017; Anderson et al., 2009; Constantino, Boswell, Berneker, & Castonguay, 2013). So what can therapists do to build these interpersonal skills and characteristics within themselves? While there is no one set way of building these skills, we believe that the framework of skills identified via FIS provides a solid foundation for training. While these FIS provide targets for training, there must also be methods for developing and practicing needed relational capacities.

Several years ago, Timothy Anderson and colleagues began a collaboration with Jeremy Safran and his laboratory to devise an integrative system for training relational skills. Jeremy Safran and colleagues had previously devised and refined a system of training known as Alliance-Focused Training (AFT; Eubanks-Carter, Muran, & Safran, 2015). AFT, developed from earlier work on brief relational therapy (BRT; Safran & Muran, 2000), attempts to build several critical processes in therapists: self-awareness, emotion regulation, and interpersonal sensitivity. AFT is a flexible framework that incorporates concrete skills along with linkages to more overarching, abstract processes. Many AFT concepts provided a natural fit to the theoretical underpinnings of FIS (i.e., the most effective therapists are those who can navigate complex, interpersonal conflicts as they occur in session).

Anderson, Safran, and colleagues developed an integrative paradigm, known in early iterations as AFT/FIS. AFT/FIS modified the scope of earlier work on AFT in a number of ways by broadening the scope of common-factors capacities covered in the training, incorporating deliberate practice elements, and utilizing the FIS as a tool for training, practice, and assessment.

Perlman, Foley, and colleagues (2019) tested the AFT/FIS paradigm by creating a brief, 1.5-hour training workshop. Sixty undergraduate students who were interested in helping/therapy-related careers signed up to participate in the study. Students were randomized to either the AFT/FIS workshop or a time-matched video demonstration of expert-delivered CBT. The researchers assessed FIS both before and after the interventions by a trained coding team who were blinded to the study conditions. There were no baseline FIS score differences between training groups. Analyses revealed a significant effect in favor of the AFT/FIS, such that participants who enrolled in the AFT/FIS training saw a more appreciable rise in FIS following their training than did participants in the expert therapy demonstration group. These results showed significant promise for a new, relational, and flexible form of therapist training that could actually enhance FIS.

The Facilitative Interpersonal Relationship Skills Training (FIRST) Program

Anderson and colleagues built on this early success by expanding their efforts to create a more comprehensive, broad-based system for therapist training, known currently as the Facilitative Interpersonal Relationship Skills Training (FIRST) program. FIRST continues the spirit of earlier AFT/FIS interventions by combining a focus on both processes and skills in a practical, applied manner. The FIRST program also more explicitly covers the full range of FIS through a broad series of training modules. Throughout the modules, a number of deliberate practice exercises are interwoven to help therapists learn and hone targeted skills (see "Deliberate Practice as a New Framework for Therapist Skill-Building" later in this chapter for more information about deliberate practice). These modules group together as verbal fluency and emotional expression; persuasion and expectations; warmth and empathy; and alliance bond capacity and ARRR. They are designed to operate sequentially, such that the modules discuss increasingly "complex" skills that build on earlier sections. In this section, we will guide you through each of the modules by providing an overview, detailing a common example of a clinical issue related to the specific skills, and describing how these skills translate into effective clinical practice.

Verbal Fluency and Emotional Expression

John, a 23-year-old first-year graduate student, is beginning his first clinical practicum experience. One of his first clients is Thomas, a 39-year-old divorced father of two. Thomas has come to therapy at the insistence of his new partner who believes that John is too hard to handle. In their first meeting, Thomas begins to explain his concerns, jumping around from states of extreme agitation, to intense worry about his relationship ending, finally ending with Thomas sobbing for the last 20 minutes of the session. John finds himself trying unsuccessfully to interject at several points throughout the session, stammering repeatedly as he tries to ask Thomas about his relationship. John feels at a loss during the session over how to connect with his new client.

Fluency and expression represent how a therapist's relational message is conveyed and understood. In high FIS responses, therapists typically speak in a way that is engaging and easy to follow, even when discussing highly volatile or challenging situations. We consider verbal fluency and emotional expression to serve as the foundational FIS. That is to say, without fluency and expression, a therapist's communication, no matter how reparative in its content, is unlikely to be well-received. By communicating in a relaxed, affectively engaged manner, therapists are able to model a level of comfort that can invite similar levels of relational involvement from clients. In emotionally charged rupture moments, high fluency and expression open a path for other skills, such as persuasion and empathy, to repair interpersonal damage. Low fluency and expression can easily be (mis)construed by clients as a lack of interest, a lack of confidence, or even a lack of competence, which has the ability to negate even the savviest of therapist responses. As such, practitioners would be wise to spend time to ensure that the physical and vocal qualities of their interventions, not just the content of those interventions, are an area of training focus. On a bodily level, showing appropriate eye contact, maintaining an open body posture, and displaying warm facial expressions can both send a positive message to clients and send internal messages to ourselves which can encourage fluent and expressive verbalizations.

For many therapists, a major barrier to effective fluency and expression is anxiety. When tense, therapists of all skill level are liable to disengage in terms of (1) our attunement/attentiveness to the process of therapy and (2) our monitoring of how we are expressing ourselves physically and verbally. When anxious or overwhelmed, a therapist can quickly be pulled out of a moment and end up demonstrating flat affect and little verbal acuity. Attentiveness to the markers of interpersonal relating cannot be overemphasized. Attentiveness to inner experience has long been observed as one of the most basic and important skills of the therapist (Anderson & Hill, 2017).

Much like our example therapist, John, clinicians wishing to build the therapeutic alliance sometimes feel "lost" in the session or may realize important moments in their therapy session several minutes after the moment has already passed. Many seasoned therapists and trainees alike have had the experience of identifying important interpersonal moments only days later when reviewing a recording of the session or when it's pointed out by a supervisor. A therapist's mind may easily become filled with thoughts and reactions, many of them important, but unfortunately, all that mental filtering can distract a therapist from perhaps the most important alliance-building skill available: full awareness to each and every moment they experience with the client.

Mindfulness may offer a unique solution for increasing awareness and, by proxy, qualities such as verbal fluency and emotional expression. Mindfulness entails the purposeful practice of placing total awareness on the here-and-now while applying a nonjudgmental mindset. For a much more complete primer on mindfulness practices and tenets, see *Full Catastrophe Living: Using the Wisdom of Your Body and Mind to Face Stress, Pain, and Illness* (Kabat-Zinn, 2013). While drawing on traditional Eastern spiritual practices, elements of mindfulness have drawn significant attention from both clinicians and psychotherapy researchers. Ryan, Safran, Doran, and Muran (2012) found that therapist trait mindfulness (particularly mindful awareness) corresponded to better client-rated alliance and outcomes in a treatment for interpersonal problems. It may be the case that higher levels of therapist awareness may correspond to better awareness of complex interpersonal processes happening in the therapy room. High levels of trait mindfulness would also aptly translate to mindfulness-in-action interventions outlined in AFT (Eubanks-Carter et al., 2015). Therapist awareness can lead to positive therapeutic interventions in the here-and-now of the session, which can improve interpersonal functioning for clients both in (and out of) the therapy room. For John, awareness may be an important skill to develop given the complexity of tracking the rapidly changing states of a client like Thomas. The use of mindfulness can be extremely helpful for therapists who are developing a greater awareness of *intra*personal states in reaction to *inter*personal input.

It is important to note that therapists do not need to have high trait levels of mindfulness to be effective at forming working alliances. Mindfulness can be treated as a "skill" and targeted for improvement in highly accessible ways. Dunn, Callahan, Swift, and Ivanovic (2013) found that 5 minutes of mindfulness practice before a session improved therapists' perceptions of their own levels of in-session presence *and* client perceptions of sessions as more effective (compared to sessions conducted without the pre-session therapist mindfulness exercise). Strong in-session engagement and presence can be considered necessary prerequisites for fluency, expression, and, ultimately, the formation of a solid client-therapist alliance.

Resolving the Clinical Example: John discusses his challenging first session with his supervisor. The pair reviews John's tape. John's supervisor notes that his client, Thomas, displayed quite a range of feelings over the course of the session. She also notices that John appeared to be highly withdrawn and closed off in his choice of posture in-session. She asked what John's experience of the session was like. This promoted John to recall the roller coaster of emotions he felt in the room: anxiety, hesitation, concern, and fear (among others). The two made a plan for John to conduct a series of deliberate practice exercises before the next session. The exercises had John review challenging moments from the tape of the prior session. While watching, John focused on increasing his attention to his own feelings as Thomas speaks. At first, John felt much of the same anxiety he experienced in the room with Thomas. John practiced providing reflections of feelings based on the taped segments and recorded as his anxiety dropped. He repeated this exercise several more times to develop greater comfort and awareness in preparation for his next session.

John also decided to conduct a brief mindful breathing exercise to help him feel more grounded and present a few minutes before his next session with Thomas. As the session begins, Thomas again jumped into a pattern of fleeting emotional states as he described an argument he had with his partner last week. A few minutes in, John catches himself as he starts to cross his arms and mentally "check-out" to cope with the frequent mood shifts in the room. He comments on his own experience of feeling overwhelmed by what's going on and asks if Thomas also has a sense of that. Thomas agrees that being overwhelmed is a good way to describe his reaction to many situations. John slows things down by opening up a conversation about the experience of being overwhelmed in the therapy space, which helps to slow down the pace, ease verbal (and non-verbal) communication, and foster a more productive working relationship.

Persuasion and Positive Expectations

Maya is a new clinician who is eager to do a good job with her clients. After reviewing literature on the wide variety of evidence-based therapies available, she has decided that she will take an eclectic approach with her new cases, combining elements of cognitive, behavioral, psychodynamic, gestalt, humanistic, feminist, and strengths-based approaches in therapy sessions. Maya believes that by including many techniques, she is more likely to figure out which approach is best suited to helping her clients. While an admirable idea, Maya's first client terminated early from therapy after feeling overwhelmed with homework assignments and a lack of understanding of where therapy was going.

Persuasion and setting positive expectations lie at the heart of therapy. Regardless of theoretical orientation or counseling style, almost all therapeutic interactions can be viewed as acts of interpersonal attitude change. Effective attitudinal, emotional, and behavioral change is a complex task with a number of components. The therapist, while not able to control all of these elements, does have an important influence. The most persuasive messages about recovery are those which are believable to clients. *Believability*, while superficially different in each case, will have common features such as a focus on specific/ unique aspects of the client's situation, building a path forward, and encouraging the client to exert active efforts to move along said path. We believe that persuasive messages are at their most effective when they are understandable and customized to each client. If successful, a persuasive message, by extension, is often helpful in building positive expectations for treatment, its outcome, and a client's sense of agency.

Examples like Maya's are extremely common among well-intentioned new clinicians. As trainees "learn the ropes" of practicing therapy, many are exposed to a variety of theories and treatment modalities in their coursework by watching video demonstrations and through reviewing empirical literature. However, the preponderance of empirical evidence supports the idea that almost all bona fide systems of therapy perform equally well for most clients (Cuijpers, van Straten, Andersson, & van Oppen, 2008; Wampold & Imel, 2015). Given a lack of clarity in which theories and specific treatment protocols are the "best," how is a clinician supposed to persuasively orient the client toward the ideal treatment?

In light of the scant group-level evidence available to inform treatment selection and implementation, we believe that this process is better considered as an individual therapist skill. Therapists must be able to appropriately match treatment techniques with specific clients in a way that feels believable and approachable with each client at each session, regardless of what those actual techniques are. In our example from the beginning of the section, Maya's eclectic systems/theory-level approach appears complex to both the client and the therapist. This complexity can easily become a distraction within session that prevents a therapist and client from forming a grounded, individualized working relationship. For new therapists, providing an appropriate level of "tailorization" can feel daunting; however, the process of selecting, framing, and implementing a treatment can be viewed as a relational act which requires the general therapist skill of persuasiveness. Indeed, the entire process of therapy has been conceptualized as an attempt to change client attitudes through persuasion (Samler, 1960). Research has found a large, positive correlation between degree of client attitude change and outcomes in therapy (Beutler, 1979).

Persuasion is already a natural, well-established component of many specific treatments. For example, early sessions of interpersonal therapy for depression establish depression as a medical illness which can be treated through an examination and alteration of interpersonal patterns (Markowitz & Weissman, 2004). In cognitive therapy, clinicians are taught to outline the interdependent relationship between thoughts, emotions, and behaviors for their clients (often using a simple triangle as a visual aid). The therapist is then tasked with convincing the client that altering biased cognitive patterns represent the most easily accessible and potent point for intervention (Beck, Rush, Shaw, & Emery, 1979). For the most part, these explanations of how psychopathology is developed, maintained, and treated are very effective: they are straightforward, understandable to most Western audiences, and offer hope for recovery. But what if a client rejects a therapist's initial rationale for treatment? Using our cognitive therapy example, what should a therapist do if a client is convinced that emotions or relationships are at the core of his or her problems?

To be a persuasive therapist, one does *not* need to take on the persona of a used car salesperson or come up with a slick sales pitch to new clients. Persuasion in therapy begins and ends with a therapeutic relationship built on mutual trust and understanding. The most persuasive therapists are often those who practice the other skills already outlined in this chapter. For example, by utilizing a personal mindfulness practice, a therapist may become more aware of subtle, interpersonal shifts as they unfold in a session. By being aware of a negative process (i.e., disruptions in the alliance), the therapist now has the opportunity to demonstrate responsiveness to the situation and offer a repair (e.g., noticing a client's uncertainty about treatment direction and offering to negotiate a change in goals or tasks).

It is also suggested that therapists have a foundational understanding of a variety of treatment approaches because different clients will have different expectations (or even demands) about what form their treatment takes. Therapists should be versed in the basics in order to appropriately respond to client preferences. It should be noted that, to be appropriately responsive, having an open conversation with a client about his or her preferences on a course of treatment will likely be more valuable to a new clinician than memorizing minute details of multiple specific treatment protocols. Meta-analytic data have shown that honoring client preferences in treatment often provides a small but significant boost to the outcome of therapy and significantly reduces the chance of early treatment dropout (Swift & Callahan, 2009).

Finally, the persuasive therapist is the one who has a genuine understanding of his or her client. The most persuasive rationales often use the client's own language and align with the client's goals. This personalized persuasion is also featured continually throughout treatment, not just in the early sessions when an overall treatment rationale is provided. Understanding clients is a continual process which can shift dramatically over the course of treatment. By consistently checking in and providing continued case conceptualization, therapists are better able to gauge their client's buy-in and agreement with the overarching plan of therapy and specific, in-session tasks. Of course, maintaining a solid agreement on treatment tasks is a central component of the therapeutic alliance. To gain a good understanding of one's clients, therapist empathy is required, which we will discuss next.

Resolving the Clinical Example: Maya is determined to do a better job with her next client. While still retaining her knowledge of various treatment modalities, Maya decides against starting her next therapy with a specific plan in place. Instead, she spends most of the first session listening to her client's concerns and attempting to understand the experiences that have brought the client to treatment. Her client, Jane, is a 25-year-old computer network technician. She was involved in a serious automobile wreck as a teen which has left her terrified of being in cars. In college, Jane was able to avoid driving with relative ease. She currently works from home and walks from place to place to get around. Jane was offered a promotion at work, but the promotion entailed travel to various offices around her area which would require driving. Jane felt awful about turning down the promotion and has come to therapy to learn how to overcome her phobia. After attentively listening to Jane's experience, Maya offers a few directions for treatment, including problem-solving, driving-related exposures, and processing

Jane's traumatic experience. Maya notes that since Jane reported wanting to overcome her fear as a primary goal, she believes that conducting a series of exposures related to driving will help Jane overcome her pattern of avoidance and anxiety most directly. Maya also briefly explains that empirical research has found exposure-based therapy to be extremely beneficial for many clients like Jane. Maya asks for Jane's opinion on directions for treatment. Jane agrees with Maya's assessment, and the two begin to plan a series of exposures for Jane to conduct.

Warmth and Empathy

Hector is a 25-year-old doctoral student clinician beginning his first external practicum experience working at an outpatient Veterans Administration (VA) medical center. While excited to work with this population, Hector is a bit anxious because he has never served in the military and knows little about the culture. Hector's first VA client, Anthony, is a gruff-looking 62-year-old combat veteran who only provides one- or two-word responses to questions in the first session. While presenting for issues of PTSD and comorbid chronic pain, Anthony appears reluctant to discuss details of his traumatic experiences with Hector. At the end of the hour, Hector feels even less confident about his ability to connect with Anthony.

Empathy represents a cornerstone of therapeutic practice. Indeed, Rogerian or client-centered therapy holds that an empathic relationship built on genuineness/congruence and unconditional positive regard can be enough to bring about clinically meaningful change (Rogers, 1951, 1957). Meta-analytic data confirm that empathy is a key process in therapy which accounts for around 10% of the variance in client outcomes (Elliott, Bohart, Watson, & Greenberg, 2011). Therapist actions can play a significant role in both gaining an empathic understanding of their clients' experiences and communicating that understanding in a relationship-fostering way.

According to MacFarlane, Anderson, and McClintock (2015), empathic interactions in therapy can be understood through three components:

1. The therapist's attunement to the client's (emotional) experience
2. The therapist's communication of said experience
3. The client's perspective on the therapist's communication.

Immediately, we can see connections to other therapist skills described in this chapter. Mindful awareness can help a therapist to attend to important information about their client's feelings. Therapists must speak persuasively, fluently, and expressively about their understanding of the client's inner world if their client is to feel genuinely understood by the therapist. All of these actions can facilitate the building of a strong therapeutic alliance. While we have attempted to reduce complex interactions into actionable concepts, it should be noted, again, that many of these skills share significant overlap and may be better viewed (from a theoretical or research perspective) as interdependent.

To build foundational skills in empathy, *helping skills* can be an excellent primer for clinicians. For a more complete introduction to helping skills, see *Helping Skills: Facilitating Exploration, Insight, and Action* (Hill & O'Brien, 2004). Helping skills refer to a series of specific, communicative actions such as reflecting a client's feelings, asking open-ended questions, and providing summaries of what someone has described. By engaging in verbal (and nonverbal) behaviors that demonstrate interest and reflect accuracy in understanding, a therapist is well on the way to building an empathic relationship. However, beyond in-session behaviors, another key component needed for empathy is *genuineness* (also referred to as "congruence" in the literature). That is to say, it is not enough for a therapist to simply provide enough reflections to help a client heal: a therapist must put in the work to genuinely understand and feel alongside their client. It is through this process of internal reflection and connection that we can form deep relationships with our clients and help them to realize important new insights.

We must also consider the way in which we convey empathy to clients. This is where the FIS of *warmth* comes into play. Similar to how a persuasive message is unlikely to be viewed as convincing if delivered in an anxious or disjointed way, an empathic communication is unlikely to be viewed as genuine or compassionate if the speaker does not also express warmth. Warmth is the expression of a genuine, caring, and accepting attitude. Warmth should be considered as a key relational skill for expressing empathy. It should also be noted that warmth does not necessarily mean that a therapist must take a warm and fuzzy approach with all cases and situations. The ideal expression of warmth will vary greatly between clients. Research shows that some clients prefer a more formal, business-like therapeutic relationship as opposed to an overtly affectively charged one (Bedi & Duff, 2009). In our clinical example, it's unlikely that Anthony would respond well to Hector if he took on a new, overtly friendly and warm tone. Instead, warmth in this case (and many others) may be better conveyed through a genuine acceptance of the client for who he is and where he is in his process of change.

So far, we've discussed components one and two of empathy. We've discussed the importance of mindfulness and genuine, internal reflection for helping us attune to our clients' experiences. We have also discussed how specific practices such as those outlined in Clara Hill's helping skills model can improve our ability to communicate about the client's experience (particularly our therapeutic understanding of it). This leaves us with component three, the client's understanding of our empathy. According to the empirical literature, this piece may be the most important for the outcome of treatment (Elliott et al., 2011). So, how should a therapist go about assessing his or her client's reception of therapist empathy?

There are a variety of methods available, the most straightforward of which involves checking in with the client. For example, after providing a summary of a client's experience, a therapist may ask a straightforward yes/no question such as, "do I have that right?" or, "is there anything I'm missing or not fully grasping?" A simple question, as a process conducted periodically throughout treatment, may work wonders for fostering an empathic relationship. Sometimes, more in-depth intervention is needed to build empathy. This is where the concept of genuineness most strongly comes into play. It may be appropriate for therapists to disclose their own feelings (even those which are "negative"), a situation they have experienced which is similar to the client, or even highlighting a difference between client and therapist in order to build empathy. By drawing attention to challenging or discrepant aspects of a healing relationship and following up with appropriate acceptance of these differences, therapists may have the opportunity to forge a deeper understanding with their clients. This technique of highlighting a difference is outlined here in the resolution to our clinical example.

Resolving the Clinical Example: Hector keeps his own discomfort in mind while heading into the second session. As he reflects on his reaction to being in the room, Hector wonders if Anthony may have also been uncomfortable, too. Hector decides to "address the elephant in the room" directly. To open the session, Hector opens up about his concerns about having trouble connecting to Anthony due to some differences between the two, particularly age and veteran identity. Hector then checks to see if his hypothesis fits Anthony's experience. To Hector's surprise, Anthony disagrees and, inspired by Hector's disclosure, admits that he was feeling a little uncomfortable opening up to Hector due to fear of judgment. Anthony barely completed high school and has been worried that Hector would think that he is unintelligent if he speaks freely. Hector thanks Anthony for his honesty and smiles as he realizes that each of them had been worried about not being seen as "good enough" by the other. Anthony chuckles in response to Hector's observation, and the two begin a more open, understanding dialogue.

Alliance Bond Capacity and Rupture Repair

Janelle is as a 19-year-old Caribbean American woman presenting for therapy, reporting symptoms of depression following a difficult transition from her home country to a rural area of the United States. Mark, her therapist, is a 29-year-old Caucasian male clinician in his first semester of clinical practice. At the end of the first session, Mark quickly checked in with Janelle about her experience during the hour. Janelle replied that she very much enjoyed therapy and was looking forward to next week. Mark had Janelle complete several brief self-report measures corresponding to Janelle's perceptions of the working alliance. Mark noticed that the alliance bond component scores were lower than expected when compared to a normative sample of outpatient clients and Mark's own view of their relationship. Mark found himself confused at the apparent discrepancy between his impression of Janelle's experience in therapy and her self-report data.

Alliance bond capacity and alliance rupture repair represent our final or most "complex" therapist FIS. While all the aforementioned skills are uniquely difficult, we consider these to be higher orders skills or capacities due to the fact that all six previously discussed FIS are often required for successful formation and reparation of the therapeutic alliance. Therapists must manage anxiety to attune to what is occurring in the room and convey persuasive and empathic messages in which vocal and nonverbal qualities match message content. It can be a tall order for therapists, especially when they are required to perform under pressure, during alliance rupture moments. Contributing to the complexity, this is an area where individual client differences can make a dramatic contribution to how we should better intervene. In this section we'll discuss ways of monitoring, assessing, and intervening effectively during key relational moments.

Looking back on our clinical examples, it should be noted that not every client is as forthcoming with difficult information as Anthony was (in our prior example in the empathy and warmth section). Sometimes, clients like Janelle, for a multitude of reasons, may not provide all information to their therapists, even when the therapist is attentive, responsive, and empathic. In situations such as these, and indeed, in a wide assortment of other clinical scenarios, the collection and analysis of client-generated data can prove invaluable for understanding and resolving relationship issues.

The use of routine feedback and progress monitoring is quickly becoming known as a best-practice in therapy. Feedback/progress monitoring can take many forms in treatment. Most often, a brief self-report measure (of process and/or outcome) is given to a client at each session. Therapists then monitor changes in the client's report over time as a measure of the effectiveness of some aspect of treatment. Overall, meta-analyses demonstrate significant efficacy for the use of feedback, especially for clients who are not demonstrating improvement or are "off-track" (Shimokawa, Lambert, & Smart 2010).

Feedback can help therapists address a number of common alliance-based concerns encountered across treatments such as:

- How/when do I check in with a client about our relationship?
- How can I combine my own perspective with my client's into a collaborative discussion?
- How can I bridge the gap between externally collected data and in-session relational processing?

Perhaps the most important result of our opening ourselves up to feedback on the working alliance is that we build a form of increased awareness into our regular practice. It's easy to assume that as therapists we can "just ask" our clients about their agreement or that we have a strong intuitive sense of our clients. However, therapists are human and prone to many social perception biases which can lead to inaccurate assessments about our cases (Hannan et al., 2005). At a minimum, using routine feedback on the working alliance provides a regular opportunity for therapists and clients to revisit their agreement on therapeutic goals and tasks. In optimal scenarios, data monitoring and feedback can assist therapists in identifying and repairing alliance ruptures.

Not all therapists repair ruptures equally well. Some therapists may overlook or deny that their actions contribute to the working alliance with their clients. Just as an athlete may explain poor performance on a variety of external or situational factors (e.g., "the sun was in my eye" or "my teammates let me down"), sometimes therapists may dwell on the client's "resistance," personality disorder diagnosis, trauma history, or string of unfortunate life events in explaining the difficulty in forming a bond or developing a collaborative plan for treatment. All of these rationales can interfere with the formation and maintenance of a working alliance.

More often, a therapist will focus on various therapeutic techniques and treatment strategies as a way to "do something" that will help the client. Techniques and strategies are a cornerstone of the "agreement on tasks" element of the working alliance. A behavioral clinician may employ exposures, a cognitive therapist may engage in cognitive restructuring, a dynamic therapist may interpret patterns that began in childhood, and a humanistic therapist may use emotional reflections. These techniques and specific strategies are the staples of the therapeutic tool belt, and many therapists focus on their implementation. In context, a predictable therapeutic approach, one that includes competently delivered techniques and strategies, can form a basis for building all of the working alliance factors of bond, collaborative tasks, and goals.

Ironically, a hyper-focus on techniques and strategies can actually disrupt the therapeutic relationship and working alliance. Perhaps the most frequent "unforced error" that therapists make is proceeding with implementing techniques and strategies without a collaborative agreement with the client. Sometimes therapists may explain their therapeutic approach without fully receiving the client's consent. More often a therapist may run afoul with the client by attaining some form agreement from the client, at least manifestly, but without the client understanding what "operations" are being planned and without fully participating and understanding those plans. Other clients may understand, but cede to the therapist, the expert in the room. The ability to empathically ascertain and understand the client's genuine reactions to the treatment is one of the most important interpersonal skills (described earlier) for forming and maintaining a therapeutic relationship.

The question of how to best implement certain interventions and at what times may be answered through a number of different strategies. The utilization of mindfulness, drawing on evidence-based treatment strategies, and demonstrating responsiveness may all be essential elements of an effective solution. Another important aspect of intervention entails directly engaging with clients about process (both positive and problematic). The next section of this chapter focuses on how therapist interpersonal strategies can be utilized to enhance alliance and outcome through direct, in-session interventions.

McClintock, Perlman, McCarrick, Anderson, and Himawan (2017) developed a novel, common factors feedback intervention to assist clinicians with addressing in-session process, including the working alliance. This feedback was structured and included, for example, the therapist providing feedback to the client about their ratings of the alliance relative to a normative sample of several hundred clients. Thus, therapists were tasked with discussing the client's perceptions of the working alliance (as well as expectations and empathy), especially at times when the working alliance was identified as being off-track via low scores. Clients who received feedback on their working alliances, outcome expectations, and empathy reported relatively faster development of positive perspectives on the working alliance over a treatment group which did not have feedback. Importantly, the presentation and discussion of feedback was relatively brief (on average, between 1 and 5 minutes in each session). Despite being a brief intervention, providing feedback was shown to have a significant impact on the formation of a strong working alliance throughout treatment.

One advantage to providing feedback on the working alliance is the encouragement of an open discussion about a construct (the working alliance). Often seen as a clinical-theoretical abstraction understood by therapists and therapy researchers, the alliance is not often the subject of direct discussions with clients. Openly sharing feedback on the working alliance is designed to provide clients with more understanding, agency, and choice in their treatment. This aligns strongly with the key FIS of building hope and positive expectations. Research has shown that client autonomy corresponds with positive alliance and treatment outcomes (Zuroff et al., 2007; Zuroff, Koestner, Moskowitz, McBride, & Bagby, 2012). By discussing crucial elements of process (i.e., the goals, tasks, and bond of the alliance; expectations about treatment; and perceptions of therapeutic empathy) clients were able to feel as though they were better understood by their therapists and more engaged/invested in the therapy because the clients saw their input being valued and actively incorporated into treatment planning and interventions.

Just as the working alliance is a pan-theoretical concept, directly discussing essential relational process can be integrated within any treatment and can be tailored to fit your genuine therapy style. Feedback in the McClintock and colleagues (2017) study was given in the context of therapists using a variety of evidence-based strategies for enhancing process. For example, when discussing alliance, clients and therapists often spoke more openly (and routinely) about the goals and tasks of treatment, allowing both parties to remain on the same page about where the therapy was heading and how the dyad was going to get there. This also provided space for open negotiation when it was determined that there was a misalignment of therapeutic goals/tasks.

Resolving the Clinical Example: Mark decided to make Janelle's low endorsement of an alliance bond a point for further exploration at session two. Mark began this second session by explaining, in straightforward terms, the concept of the alliance, and he provided a basic visualization of Janelle's data compared to a normative sample. When he got to the bond section of the feedback, Mark disclosed that his knowledge of Caribbean culture was extremely limited, and he asked Janelle if it would be worthwhile to focus therapy on understanding Janelle's experiences from this culture and how they related to her transition into the United States. Mark also disclosed minority aspects of his own identity as being impactful in his own day-to-day life as a way to highlight areas of both commonality and contrast in the therapy dyad. Janelle agreed that culture and identity would be important to discuss. Mark ensured that much of the remaining therapy allowed Janelle space to describe her culture, what it meant to her, how she felt out of place following her move, and her lack of connection to others in the United States. At the end of treatment, she described the overall therapy experience as extremely helpful and reported significant increases in later administered measures of alliance (as well as dramatic reductions in depressive symptoms).

Deliberate Practice as a New Framework for
Therapist Skill-Building

In many traditional forms of therapy training, novice therapists may be provided feedback, typically in supervision, on a clinical interaction they had days or even weeks ago. Given the significant variability that comes with client interactions, the feedback or suggestions given may not apply to future sessions. As such, trainees may not have the opportunity to conduct important practice of key interpersonal skills. Deliberate practice has been identified as a key mechanism by which therapists are able to build skills over time.

Miller, Hubble, and Chow (2017) provide a four-pronged definition of deliberate practice which includes (1) a targeted, systematic approach to improving performance; (2) a mentor or trainer to guide the process; (3) regular, immediate feedback on the development of targeted skills; and (4) repeated practice and refinement in skill utilization. Research by Chow and colleagues (2015) found that therapists who put more time and effort into practicing areas of weakness/specific skills, such as reviewing their session tapes, reliably had the best outcomes compared to peers. Deliberate practice can provide a strong foundational approach to developing alliance skills. For example, if a trainee has access to recordings of their sessions, they may be able to review the tape for a challenging segment and repeatedly focus on tapping into their emotional experience (as they watch the tape) using the recording as a stimulus. A trainee could also review a challenging segment or moment of alliance rupture and utilize deliberate practice to rethink their response and come up with alternative repair attempts. There are a vast array of ways in which deliberate practice could be incorporated in line with the training strategies which we discuss later in the chapter. Deliberate practice can be completed alone or with a mentor. For a comprehensive introduction to deliberate practice, see *Deliberate Practice for Psychotherapists: A Guide to Improving Clinical Effectiveness* (Rousmaniere, 2016).

Summary

To summarize, the intersection of therapist skills and alliance development may not be best understood through learning to/adhering to specific treatment protocols. Instead, best practices for building the working alliance involve the following:

1. Focus training efforts primarily on the development of key interpersonal skills which help therapists navigate critical relational markers or ruptures in the alliance.

2. Consider integrating mindfulness in one's day-to-day life and clinical practice.

3. Have a flexible background in diverse, evidence-based approaches (e.g., familiarizing yourself with basic helping skills and understanding the basics of multiple therapeutic modalities) in order to flexibly meet the treatment needs of each client.

4. Gather feedback, and be receptive to modifying interventions in the face of client-generated feedback/progress monitoring. Feedback is typically best employed as a way to open in-session negotiations of the therapeutic relationship or other aspects of treatment process.

5. Focus on implementation in a way that fits with your style and the specific context of the client as it unfolds at that moment.

6. Utilize deliberate practice to assess and develop interpersonal skills throughout one's career. Deliberate practice can be an excellent, complementary training modality for any of the therapist FIS discussed in this chapter.

We understand that no clinician is perfect with all clients at all moments. The aforementioned principles should be considered an aspirational integration of various concepts including mindfulness and alliance-focused strategies, collecting data, understanding treatment modalities, and engaging in deliberate practice in order to be flexible, develop skills, and have tools at the ready for a variety of clinical situations. To properly integrate these complex concepts, we suggest that trainees take a deliberate practice mindset in their development. This mindset entails several key ideas (Chow et al., 2015):

1. Treat improvement as a value and a process, not an attainable goal.

2. Focus on continuous improvement throughout one's career—not just in graduate school.

3. Routinely target specific skills, *especially* around weak points.

4. Learn to appreciate (if not enjoy) challenging aspects of therapy. These moments provide some of the most valuable lessons for our development as therapists.

5. Seek out supervision and regular feedback on areas of growth.

Ultimately, learning to grow and maintain strong alliances with clients is a challenging interpersonal process. While the development of any given alliance will be unique to each therapist–client dyad, the foundational practices and concepts highlighted in this chapter may provide a solid basis for therapists to be broadly responsive, flexible, and effective in fostering alliances with any client.

References

Anderson, T., Crowley, M. E. J., Patterson, C. L., & Heckman, B. D. (2012). The influence of supervision on manual adherence and therapeutic processes. *Journal of Clinical Psychology, 68*, 972–988.

Anderson, T., Crowley, M. J., Himawan, L., Holmberg, J., Uhlin, B. (2015). Therapist facilitative interpersonal skills and training status: A randomized clinical trial on alliance and outcome. *Psychotherapy Research, 26*, 511–529.

Anderson, T., & Hill, C. E. (2017). The role of therapist skills in therapist effectiveness. In L. G. Castonguay & C. E Hill (Eds.), *How and why are some therapists better than others? Understanding therapist effects* (pp. 139–157). Washington DC: American Psychological Association.

Anderson, T., McClintock, A. S., Himawan, L., Song, X., & Patterson, C. L. (2016). A prospective study of therapist facilitative interpersonal skills as a predictor of treatment outcome. *Journal of Consulting and Clinical Psychology, 84*, 57–66. doi:10.1037/ccp0000060.

Anderson, T., Ogles, B. M., Patterson, C. L., Lambert, M. J., & Vermeersch, D. A. (2009). Therapist effects: Facilitative interpersonal skills as a predictor of therapist success. *Journal of Clinical Psychology, 65*, 755–768.

Anderson, T., Ogles, B. M., & Weis, A. T. (1999). Creative use of interpersonal skills in building a therapeutic alliance. *Journal of Constructivist Psychology, 12*, 313–330.

Anderson, T., & Strupp, H. H. (2015). Training in time-limited dynamic psychotherapy: A systematic comparison of pre- and post-training cases treated by one therapist. *Psychotherapy Research, 25*, 595–611.

Baldwin, S. A., & Imel, Z. E. (2013). Therapist effects: Findings and methods. In M. J. Lambert (Ed.), *Bergin and Garfield's handbook of psychotherapy and behavior change* (6th ed., pp. 258–297). New York: Wiley.

Beck, A. T., Rush, A. J., Shaw, B. F., & Emery, G. (1979). *Cognitive therapy of depression.* New York: Guilford Press.

Bedi, R. P., & Duff, C. T. (2009). Prevalence of counselling alliance type preferences across two samples. *Canadian Journal of Counselling, 43*, 152–164.

Beutler, L. E. (1979). Values, beliefs, religion and the persuasive influence of psychotherapy. *Psychotherapy: Theory, Research & Practice, 16*, 432–440.

Bordin, E. S. (1979). The generalizability of the psychoanalytic concept of the working alliance. *Psychotherapy: Theory, Research & Practice, 16*, 252–260.

Chow, D. L., Miller, S. D., Seidel, J. A., Kane, R. T., Thornton, J. A., & Andrews, W. P. (2015). The role of deliberate practice in the development of highly effective psychotherapists. *Psychotherapy, 52*, 337–345. doi:10.1037/pst0000015

Constantino, M., Boswell, J., Berneker, S., & Castonguay, L. (2013). Context-responsive psychotherapy integration as a framework for a unified clinical science: Conceptual and empirical considerations. *Journal of Unified Psychotherapy and Clinical Science, 2*, 1–20.

Constantino, M. J., Morrison, N. R., Coyne, A. E., & Howard, T. (2017). Exploring therapeutic alliance training in clinical and counseling psychology graduate programs. *Training and Education in Professional Psychology, 11*, 219–226.

Crits-Christoph, P., Gibbons, M. B. C., Crits-Christoph, K., Narducci, J., Schamberger, M., & Gallop, R. (2006). Can therapists be trained to improve their alliances? A preliminary study of alliance-fostering psychotherapy. *Psychotherapy Research, 16*, 268–281.

Cuijpers, P., van Straten, A., Andersson, G., & van Oppen, P. (2008). Psychotherapy for depression in adults: A meta-analysis of comparative outcome studies. *Journal of Consulting and Clinical Psychology, 76,* 909–922.

Dunn, R., Callahan, J. L., Swift, J. K., & Ivanovic, M. (2013). Effects of pre-session centering for therapists on session presence and effectiveness. *Psychotherapy Research, 23,* 78–85.

Elliot, R. Bohart, A. C., Watson, J. C., & Greenberg, L. S. (2011). Empathy. *Psychotherapy, 48,* 43–49.

Eubanks-Carter, C., Muran, J. C., & Safran, J. D. (2015). Alliance-focused training. *Psychotherapy, 52,* 169–173.

Henry, W. P., Strupp, H. H., Butler, S. F., Schacht, T. E., & Binder, J. L. (1993). Effects of training in time-limited dynamic psychotherapy: Changes in therapist behavior. *Journal of Consulting and Clinical Psychology, 61,* 434–440.

Hannan, C., Lambert, M. J., Harmon, C., Nielsen, S. L., Smart, D. W., & Shimokawa, K. (2005). A lab test and algorithms for identifying clients at risk for treatment failure. *Journal of Clinical Psychology, 61,* 155–163.

Hatcher, R. L., & Barends, A. W. (2006). How a return to theory could help alliance research. *Psychotherapy: Theory, Research, Practice, Training, 43,* 292–299.

Hill, C. E., & O'Brien, K. M. (2004). *Helping skills: Facilitating exploration, insight, and action.* Washington, DC: American Psychological Association.

Kabat-Zinn, J. (2013). *Full catastrophe living (revised edition): Using the wisdom of your body and mind to face stress, pain, and illness.* New York: Bantam.

Laska, K. M., Smith, T. L., Wislocki, A., Minami, T., & Wampold, B. E. (2013). Uniformity of evidence based treatments in practice? Therapist effects in the delivery of cognitive processing therapy for PTSD. *Journal of Counseling Psychology, 60,* 31–41. http://dx.doi.org/10.1037/a0031294

MacFarlane, P., Anderson, T., & McClintock, A. S. (2015). The early formation of the working alliance from the client's perspective: A qualitative study. *Psychotherapy, 52,* 363–372.

Markowitz, J. C., & Weissman, M. M. (2004). Interpersonal psychotherapy: Principles and applications. *World Psychiatry, 3,* 136–139.

McClintock, A. S., Perlman, M. R., McCarrick, S., Anderson, T., & Himawan, L. (2017). Enhancing psychotherapy process with common factors feedback: A randomized clinical trial. *Journal of Counseling Psychology, 64,* 247–260.

Miller, S. D., Hubble, M. A., & Chow, D. L. (2017). Professional development: From oxymoron to reality. In T. Rousmaniere, R. K. Goodyear, S. D. Miller, & B. E. Wampold (Eds.), *The cycle of excellence: Using deliberate practice to improve supervision and training* (pp. 23–47). New York: John Wiley.

Perlman, M. R., Foley, V. K., Finkelstein, J., Anderson, T., Mimnaugh, S., David, K. C., Gooch, C. V., . . . Safran, J. D. (2019). *Results from a preliminary test of AFT/FIS.* Manuscript submitted for publication.

Rogers, C. R. (1951). *Client-centered therapy: Its current practice, implications, and theory.* Boston: Houghton Mifflin.

Rogers, C. R. (1957). The necessary and sufficient conditions of therapeutic personality change. *Journal of Consulting Psychology, 21,* 95–103.

Rousmaniere, T. (2016). *Deliberate practice for psychotherapists: A guide to improving clinical effectiveness.* New York: Routledge.

Ryan, A., Safran, J. D., Doran, J. M., & Muran, J. C. (2012). Therapist mindfulness, alliance and treatment outcome. *Psychotherapy Research, 22*, 289–297.

Safran, J. D., & Muran, J. C. (2000). *Negotiating the therapeutic alliance: A relational treatment guide*. New York: Guilford Press.

Samler, J. (1960). Change in values: A goal in counseling. *Journal of Counseling Psychology, 7*, 32–39.

Shimokawa, K., Lambert, M. J., & Smart, D. W. (2010). Enhancing treatment outcome of patients at risk of treatment failure: Meta-analytic and mega-analytic review of a psychotherapy quality assurance system. *Journal of Consulting and Clinical Psychology, 78*, 298–311. doi:10.1037/a0019247

Smith-Hansen, L., Constantino, M. J., Piselli, A., & Remen, A. L. (2011). Preliminary results of a video-assisted psychotherapist workshop in alliance strategies. *Psychotherapy, 48*, 148–162.

Stiles, W. B., Honos-Webb, L., & Surko, M. (1998). Responsiveness in psychotherapy. *Clinical Psychology: Science and Practice, 5*, 439–458.

Swift, J. K., & Callahan, J. L. (2009). The impact of client treatment preferences on outcome: A meta-analysis. *Journal of Clinical Psychology, 65*, 368–381.

Wampold, B. E., & Brown, G. S. (2005). Estimating variability in outcomes attributable to therapists: A naturalistic study of outcomes in managed care. *Journal of Consulting and Clinical Psychology, 73*, 914–923. http://dx.doi.org/10.1037/0022-006X.73.5.914

Wampold, B. E., & Imel, Z. E. (2015). *The great psychotherapy debate: The evidence for what makes psychotherapy work* (2nd edition). New York: Routledge.

Wampold, B. E., Mondin, G. W., Moody, M., Stich, F., Benson, K., & Ahn, H. N. (1997). A meta-analysis of outcome studies comparing bona fide psychotherapies: Empirically, "all must have prizes." *Psychological Bulletin, 122*, 203–215.

Webb, C. A., DeRubeis, R. J., & Barber, J. P. (2010). Therapist adherence/competence and treatment outcome: A meta-analytic review. *Journal of Consulting and Clinical Psychology, 78*, 200–211. http://dx.doi.org/10.1037/a0018912

Zuroff, D. C., Koestner, R., Moskowitz, D. S., McBride, C., & Bagby, R. M. (2012). Therapist's autonomy support and patient's self-criticism predict motivation during brief treatments for depression. *Journal of Social and Clinical Psychology, 31*, 903–932.

Zuroff, D. C., Koestner, R., Moskowitz, D. S., McBride, C., Marshall, M., & Bagby, M. R. (2007). Autonomous motivation for therapy: A new common factor in brief treatments for depression. *Psychotherapy Research, 17*, 137–147. doi:10.1080/10503300600919380

4

Setting Goals and Tasks in the Working Alliance

Georgiana Shick Tryon

It seems obvious that during psychotherapy, both patient and therapist are in agreement on the goals of therapy and the methods to achieve them. Indeed, there is both theoretical (Bordin, 1979) and empirical (Tryon, Birch, & Verkuilen, 2018) support for the conceptualization of therapist–client agreement on the goals and tasks of therapy as a component of the working alliance that relates to positive psychotherapy outcomes. In practice, however, some therapists and patients do not agree on the goals that they are working toward or how to achieve them (Swift & Callahan, 2008; Zane et al., 2005), thus compromising their work together and sometimes leading to patients' premature termination. In some instances, because of the type of therapy or the type of therapists, goals are never discussed nor are tasks specified.

This chapter aims to facilitate the development of positive working alliances by providing practitioners with skills to assist in collaborating with patients to set attainable therapy goals and to choose ways to achieve those goals. Specifically, the chapter presents suggestions for determining the patient's problem and what life changes the patient wants to make. Next, the chapter discusses collaborative goal setting focusing on attainable goals based on patients' wishes. Following this, the chapter describes the collaborative formulation of treatment plans to achieve goals. Finally, the chapter concludes with a discussion of therapy termination from a goal perspective.

Assessing the Patient's Problem

One might think that it would be easy to achieve therapist–patient goal consensus, but accounts by real-life patients indicate that this is not always the case (Feltham, Martin, Walker, & Harris, 2018). Often therapists will acknowledge that patients have problems and meet with them regularly with little direction concerning where treatment is going or how or when it will end.

The extent to which goal consensus can be quickly and easily achieved varies with each patient. Indeed, some individuals present with relatively well-defined concerns that, when left unaddressed, might negatively affect their lives. For example, a university freshman enrolled in a class that requires him to deliver a speech may seek help for his public speaking anxiety. A businesswoman who takes a position that requires extensive travel may enter therapy to overcome a fear of flying. It is not difficult to imagine achieving goal consensus with either of these patients. Others, however, seek help for concerns that are less well-defined. For instance, a recently divorced woman may complain of sadness and anxiety. Still others enter therapy because of outside pressures rather than their own desires. For example, an employer may refer an employee for workplace problems and make continued employment contingent upon therapy attendance. Research suggests that collaborative goal consensus will facilitate better therapy outcomes for each of these patients (Tryon et al., 2018). Collaborative determination of goals and tasks is at the heart of Bordin's (1979) formulation of the working alliance.

Active Listening and Questioning

Therapy begins with a determination of the patient's problem to answer the question, "What brings you to therapy?" There are several reasons that patients need to tell the story of their concerns. It is important to establish a good working relationship with patients, and this begins with therapists' including them as partners by seeking and listening to patients' input. To determine therapeutic goals, it is important for both therapists and patients to have a clear understanding of the problem. Although some patients' problems, such as the concerns about public speaking and airline travel just presented, may seem apparent, they may be more complex than initially thought. Patients have been living with their problems and are the best source of information about them; however, sometimes patients are not themselves entirely clear about why they are seeking help. They may be troubled, but, to establish clear goals, the exact focus of their distress needs clarification.

Thus, the initial session, or sessions, of psychotherapy focuses on exploration of patients' reasons for seeking help. This exploratory phase of therapy is best informed by a humanistic therapeutic orientation such as that espoused by Rogers (1957). Therapists adopt a warm, empathic, and accepting posture that is free of preconceptions and open to learning, which facilitates patient sharing. Therapists pay close attention to what their patients tell them and encourage them to talk openly about their concerns. Hill (2014) provides descriptions and detailed instructions of specific helping skills that therapists can use to explore patients' concerns.

Active listening implies focusing attention on patients and what they are saying. Leaning toward the patient, making eye contact, and nodding one's head are nonverbal ways of showing therapist attention to the patients' stories. Therapists' use of open questions (i.e., questions that ask patients to elaborate) rather than closed questions (i.e., questions that can be answered with a "yes" or "no") encourages patients to explore concerns. Therapists' restatement of what patients say, as well as reflection of patients' feelings, facilitates further elaboration of their concerns.

Notice how the therapist uses restatements and reflection of feelings in the exploratory interview for the imaginary student (Jamal) who has to give a speech.

THERAPIST: [Leaning toward the patient and making eye contact.] Tell me about what brings you here today.

JAMAL: I'm a freshman and I signed up for this course that has you give a speech that counts as half of your final grade. I figured it would be a tough course, so I'd get it out of the way early. But I may have bitten off more than I can chew.

THERAPIST: You seem to be regretting your choice.

JAMAL: In some ways I do, but if I drop the course, I'd only have to face taking it again.

THERAPIST: So just thinking about the course, whether you take it now or take it later, makes you anxious.

JAMAL: Every time I have to speak in public it freaks me out, and having a speech count for so much makes me even more upset.

THERAPIST: Sounds like you'd like to have a different approach to this course.

JAMAL: For sure, I just can't go around upset about it all the time. I want to enjoy college.

Following this exchange, the therapist continues to use her active listening skills to explore Jamal's concerns about the upcoming speech. In response to her questions and reflections, Jamal details his worries about his course grade and speech preparation and presentation. At the end of the session, the therapist summarizes what he has told her and invites him to provide additions and corrections.

The therapist employs the same skills in the exploratory sessions for the imaginary recently divorced woman (Jill), but her story unfolds over several sessions.

THERAPIST: [Leaning toward the patient and making eye contact.] What brings you here today?

JILL: I got divorced 2 months ago, and I just don't seem myself anymore. I am so upset all the time that I can barely sleep or concentrate on anything.

THERAPIST: Seems like you've been through a lot.

JILL: Indeed I have. I didn't think our marriage was going that badly. Then one day, he comes home and announces that he wants a divorce because things aren't working out like he planned. Wish he would have shared his plan with me before he decided to throw in the towel.

THERAPIST: Sounds like you're angry at him for not including you as a partner in your marriage.

JILL: You're right. I believe that marriage is a partnership and that things can be worked out in that partnership. Now, here I am, left all alone.

Over the next several sessions, the therapist uses reflection of feelings, closed questions, and restatements to listen actively to Jill's story in a warm, nonjudgmental way. The therapist provides summaries of what Jill has said at the end of each session.

Transitioning from "Why Are You Here?" to "What Would You Like to Change?"

After therapists have heard patients' stories, they summarize what patients have told them and ask for clarifications and additions. Then therapists work collaboratively with patients to determine what changes patients would like to make. During the course of this transition phase, patients may identify several things that they would like to change about their lives. Therapists help them to clarify which of these changes they would like to work on first.

THERAPIST: It appears that you have several concerns about your upcoming speech. You seem to lack confidence in your ability to prepare adequately and are concerned that classmates and particularly the instructor will judge what you present badly. You also worry that you'll be too nervous to give a good presentation and that others will feel sorry for you or laugh at you. You seem concerned that other students will find fault with your appearance as well.

JAMAL: That sums it up pretty well.

THERAPIST: We can work on each of these things, but perhaps there is one thing that we could focus on first.

JAMAL: I can't see myself being able to pull this off unless I am more confident about getting up there and having people not laugh at me. I guess I need to believe that I can speak in public without practically dying of anxiety.

THERAPIST: So you would like to begin by focusing on changing how you feel when you make a speech.

In this next case, the therapist summarizes what Jill has told her about her concerns. Notice that Jill expresses appreciation for the opportunity to tell her story without being judged. The therapist's nonjudgmental approach has facilitated Jill's understanding of her concerns and what she'd like to change.

THERAPIST: Over the past three meetings, you have told me your story. The break-up of your marriage has left you angry and concerned about how you will cope on your own, both financially and psychologically. You have doubts about your ability to make decisions that are in your best interests.

JILL: I am grateful for the opportunity to tell you how I feel. It helps me to put some of the issues in my life into perspective. My friends have given me a lot of advice and some of them have been very sympathetic. But others say that I should just get over it and live my life. However, I'm not sure what my life should be. In talking to you, I realize that I have always had others tell me what is good for me, including my ex-husband.

THERAPIST: It seems that you are saying that you'd like to be more accepting of yourself.

JILL: I don't believe in myself, in my own judgment. I have been too willing to do what others want for me rather than to have asked myself what I want. What this has gotten me is a bad marriage and some friends that are not always on my side. I want to be on my side.

THERAPIST: It sounds like we can start working on helping you be on your side.

Collaborative Goal Setting in Patients' Best Interests

The therapist collaborated with Jamal and Jill to decide on the general goals of their treatment. The goals they decided on appear to be in their best interests. Jamal may have a better chance of obtaining a good grade on his speech if he is less anxious about delivering it. Jill might make better life choices if she becomes more self-accepting. Sometimes, however, patients espouse goals that are clearly not in their best interests.

Finding Helpful Rather Than Harmful Goals

Certain goals may be harmful, even life-threatening, to patients. For example, if a patient with anorexia nervosa wants to lose more weight, this would certainly not be a goal that her therapist should agree to. Although disagreeing with a patient's goal is not what comes to mind when one thinks of collaborative goal setting, it is important to keep the patient from harm. An examination of the patient's motive for choosing to lose weight could lead to a less harmful goal. The therapist could ask, "Why is it important for you to lose more weight?" The patient might then provide reasons for doing so, and the reasons may yield a less harmful goal, such as the desire to have friends or the wish to feel good about oneself. The therapist could say, "we can work together to help you develop friendships in ways that do not include losing weight." Often it can take several sessions of active empathic listening for the patient to switch to a less harmful goal. At times, however, the patient will not adopt a different goal. Patients who have eating disorders sometimes have to be hospitalized.

Suicidal clients also need to be dissuaded from self-harm. When patients tell therapists that they are thinking about suicide, therapists should assess the danger involved by questioning patients about the seriousness of their intent, the means they have to carry out the intent, past suicidal thoughts and behaviors, and sources of support available to them. If patients are in immediate danger of suicide, they may have to be hospitalized. Therapists may develop a contract, which includes people and places to contact, with patients who are in less immediate danger. It is particularly important for therapists to consult supervisors and colleagues when seeing patients who are inclined toward life-threatening behaviors, such as anorexia and suicide.

The therapist's goal is to convince patients to adopt a different goal than suicide, and this begins by asking them why they want to kill themselves. Their answers may lead to less harmful goals.

Patients with eating disorders or suicidal thoughts are not the only ones who may have goals that are more harmful than helpful. Sometimes patients who do not come to therapy voluntarily voice goals that may be harmful to themselves or to others. These patients may not believe they need therapy, and they may be angry at the people who referred them. They may want to change other people rather than work on their own problems. For example, the imaginary employee referred for workplace problems may voice anger at his employer who made continued employment contingent on therapy attendance.

THERAPIST: I know that you don't want to be here and that you are angry with your boss for saying that you have to be here or lose your job. Perhaps there are things that we might work on to help you change your situation.

JIM: My boss should be fired. Can you get my boss fired? That would help a lot.

THERAPIST: I can't do that, but if you tell me what has been happening at work, we may be able to determine ways to help you keep your job.

JIM: My boss is always sneaking around, checking up on me, and if I even do one measly little thing, he gets upset.

THERAPIST: It seems you feel unfairly singled out for some reason. What things upset him?

JIM: Oh, there's this guy who works next to me, and I kinda joke around with him, but he doesn't take it that way and the boss gets pissed. The guy picks on me, too, but the boss doesn't punish him, he just threatens to fire me.

THERAPIST: If you had a better relationship with this co-worker, do you think your boss might back off?

JIM: I'm not sure, maybe.

THERAPIST: Since you are supposed to attend our sessions, we could use them to explore some things you might do to improve your work relationship situation.

JIM: I guess. Sounds better than doing nothing. You know, just sitting here.

Although Jim has some reluctance about participating in therapy, he does seem willing to give it a try. Others who attend therapy against their wishes may not be so inclined. They may even threaten violence against the persons who referred them. It is important for therapists to take such threats seriously and consult with supervisors and colleagues. It is the therapist's duty to warn and protect individuals who are targets of violent threats. This may include notifying law enforcement.

Like Jim, patients who are self-referred sometimes come to therapy seeking to change others rather than themselves. Therapists cannot collaborate with patients to change people who are not their patients, so changing others is not a helpful goal. If patients concentrate on changing others, they lose the opportunity to change their own behavior for the better, and the problematic situations with others may even get worse. Jim's wish to have the therapist get his boss fired is beyond what therapy can achieve. If Jim attains the goal of having a better relationship with his co-worker, his boss may behave in a more positive manner toward him, but this outcome is not guaranteed. Jim and his therapist can only work toward their agreed upon goal.

Working Together to Set Attainable Goals

Unfortunately, for one reason or another, even helpful goals may not always be attainable. Sometimes patients find that the work needed to achieve their goals is too difficult. Sometimes they lack the resources (e.g., support system, time, money) to enable them to reach their goals. It is important to set goals that patients have reasonable expectations of achieving.

Exploring the Attainability of Various Goal Types

Berking, Grosse Holtforth, Jacobi, and Kröner-Herwig (2005) examined the treatment goals of more than 2,770 patients and found that goals that were re-lated to patients' well-being (such as learning to relax and improving leisure activities) yielded better treatment outcomes than did more existential goals (such as coming to terms with one's past). They recommend that therapists use the results of their research in collaborative goal setting to motivate patients to choose more attainable goals. Our imaginary patients Jamal and Jill have chosen goals (being more relaxed while giving a speech, achieving self-acceptance) that are high on Berking et al.'s list of attainable goals. According to their research, well-being goals are most attainable followed by interpersonal goals, personal growth goals, and symptom-related goals, with existential issues having the lowest average goal attainment.

Intrinsic goals (goals that are themselves rewarding) are generally associated with better therapy outcomes than are *extrinsic goals* (goals that are imposed by external pressures) (Michalak & Grosse Holtforth, 2006). Patients are more motivated to attain goals that are consistent with their wishes for themselves. Goals that address patients' sense of well-being and life satisfaction, such as Jill's goal of being more self-accepting, are intrinsically motivating.

In contrast, extrinsic goals are frequently more grudgingly pursued and may not be achieved, such as Jim's goal of improving his relationship with a co-worker in hopes that his boss will not fire him. He does not particularly like his co-worker or his boss. His therapy attendance is imposed externally by the boss. The goal he marginally accepts is just "better than doing nothing." Keeping his job may or may not provide sufficient motivation for Jim to attain his relationship goal. Similarly, someone in treatment for alcoholism because of external pres-sure from family or employer may not be motivated to finish the treatment. On the other hand, a person who decides on his own that his life would be better if he enters treatment for alcohol abuse would be more motivated to complete treatment successfully because he does not feel pressured by others but instead perceives himself as a person who should not abuse alcohol.

Approach goals (goals that focus on moving toward a more desirable state) are generally associated with more improvement than *avoidance goals* (goals that focus on avoiding a negative state) (Elliot & Church, 2002). Jill's goal of self-acceptance is an approach goal; so is Jamal's goal of being more relaxed while speaking in public.

The therapist's framing of Jim's goal as improving his relationship with his co-worker is also an approach goal. It is a more achievable than a goal that would suggest that Jim avoid "teasing" his co-worker. Avoidance goals focus on staying away from something negative. This is often difficult to do because situations and feelings to be avoided inevitably arise. Avoidance goals do not provide patients with something to replace the feeling or behavior that is avoided. If Jim successfully avoids teasing his co-worker, what behavior might he substitute? Will he "tease" someone else instead? Will he become even angrier at his boss?

In contrast, approach goals provide patients with something positive to work toward. As patients get closer to achieving their approach goals, their motivation for continued progress increases. In contrast, "trying to avoid something is inherently problematic because it requires us to call to mind the thing we want to avoid, hence making it more salient" (Cooper, 2018, p. 42).

Reworking Less Attainable Goals to Make Them More Attainable

The preceding section discussed how therapists might rework goals for suicidal patients and patients with anorexia. Other less life-threatening goals that may be difficult to achieve can be reworked in collaboration with patients to facilitate their attainability. Often avoidance goals can be reframed as approach goals in a manner provided by the following example.

Maria describes herself as a perfectionist who is highly self-critical. She has a high-stress job in business that she likes, but she finds that her self-criticism adds to an already stressful occupation. Believing that she would be happier and more relaxed if she were less critical of herself, she undertook her own self-improvement campaign. When this proved to be more harmful than helpful, she decided to enter psychotherapy.

MARIA: So I try to catch myself every time I am self-critical. I've become super vigilant.

THERAPIST: How has that been working for you?

MARIA: Not well. I seem to be even more self-critical now than I was before I started this process. Every time I find myself being self-critical, I criticize myself for criticizing myself. Then I wonder if I'll ever be able to stop doing this.

THERAPIST: So you're starting to feel hopeless about breaking the cycle of self-criticism.

MARIA: Absolutely. Clearly, I need help. I am just making myself worse.

THERAPIST: Perhaps you might look at your problem in another way.

MARIA: How can I possibly do that?

THERAPIST: If you were able to stop criticizing yourself, how do you envision yourself being?

MARIA: Well, I wouldn't be so negative about myself. I'd be happier and not focus on what I am doing wrong all the time.

THERAPIST: So you're saying that currently you aren't very kind to yourself, and, if you were kinder to yourself, you'd be happier. If your goal was to be kinder to yourself, you could focus on the things you do well rather than looking for things you don't do so well.

MARIA: Yes. Perhaps that's what I need to learn to do. Focusing on my weaknesses led to more weaknesses.

THERAPIST: Instead of focusing on detecting self-criticism, focusing on what you do well might allow you to see the positives rather than the negatives.

Sometimes patients enter psychotherapy because of life dissatisfactions as a result of pursuing extrinsic rather than intrinsic goals. For example, Fred is a first-year medical student who came to therapy reporting depression. He excelled as a pre-med undergraduate, even though he was not that interested in his courses.

FRED: I thought that once I got to medical school, things would be different. I'd be learning real doctor stuff, and maybe I'd like that, but I don't.

THERAPIST: Sounds like you're rethinking what you want to do with your life.

FRED: I can't do that. I'm supposed to be a doctor. My family is counting on me. My dad would be so pissed if he even knew I was talking to you about this.

THERAPIST: You seem to feel under a great deal of pressure.

Fred recounts how he is the first person in his family to attend college, and how his family decided that he should become a doctor because doctors make lots of money. However, he never wanted to be a doctor. Thus, Fred's extrinsic goal appears to be based on what he believes his family wants. It may be that his belief is correct, but he is afraid to talk to them about this.

> THERAPIST: It is very hard to have a career doing something you don't like. Here you are in just your first year of medical school, and you're already feeling sad and depressed. Perhaps there is some other career you'd like to pursue.
>
> FRED: Actually, I think I'd kinda like to be a teacher. I had some really wonderful teachers in high school, and I often thought I'd really like to do what they do. Only thing is, they don't make much money.
>
> THERAPIST: Your choice seems to be between making money as a doctor and having a fulfilling job.
>
> FRED: I would really like to have a fulfilling job even if I didn't make a lot of money, but I don't think my family would support this.

Thus, Fred's goal is to allow himself to pursue an intrinsic goal rather than the extrinsic goal he believes his family wants.

Determining a Course of Action

After therapists have worked together with patients to set goals, they need to collaborate with them to establish treatment tasks that will help patients achieve these goals. As with goal consensus, consensus on tasks requires patients' input. If patients do not believe in or are not willing to undertake certain tasks, their goals may not be reached, and patients will not receive the help they sought. Active listening skills are important to determine the course of action that is agreeable to each patient. Therapists also need to provide information about the task choices that are available to patients. Therapists' theoretical orientation often affects the tasks that are presented. For example, a therapist who is trained in psychodynamic psychotherapy would generally not suggest behavioral tasks to achieve goals.

Collaboratively Formulating Treatment Plans to Achieve Goals

Jamal's goal is to be less anxious while giving a speech that will determine half his course grade, but he is also concerned about writing a good speech. His therapist refers him to the college writing center in order to help him construct the speech, and Jamal's instructor agrees to review drafts of the speech before he gives it.

Jamal's therapist has a behavioral theoretical orientation, and she and Jamal set the tasks of therapy within this framework.

THERAPIST: To help you to be more relaxed during your speech, we can first develop a hierarchy or list of speech situations that are progressively more anxiety provoking for you. Then you will go through each step in the hierarchy in a real-life situation until you feel very little anxiety. We have an empty classroom here that we can use for that purpose.

JAMAL: How will that hierarchy part go?

THERAPIST: The hierarchy will start with speech situations that make you feel just a little anxiety and progress to situations that make you feel the most anxious. For instance, how do you feel when you enter a room where public speaking occurs?

JAMAL: If I'm not giving a speech, I don't feel that anxious. If I know I'll be speaking, I feel a little more anxious.

THERAPIST: Okay, so the hierarchy will start with the situation in which you feel the least anxious, like the one you just identified, and end with the situation in which you feel the most anxious, which I think will be delivering your speech.

JAMAL: Where does the room come in?

THERAPIST: You will go through each hierarchy step while you are in the room until you feel much less anxiety. After the first step, you'll go to step two. The final step will be giving your speech to an audience. How do you feel about this approach?

JAMAL: It sounds good to me. Will I have enough time to do all this?

THERAPIST: I think so. You came for help right at the beginning of the semester. We have 13 weeks left. If needed, we can meet twice a week.

Jamal and the therapist next construct the hierarchy. The therapist records the steps that Jamal provides from least to most anxiety causing. She reads the steps back to him several times, and he and she collaborate to rearrange and revise them.

Jill's therapist has a psychodynamic orientation that stresses insight as a task to achieve therapy goals.

THERAPIST: It seems that you have not been accepting of yourself for quite a while. It might help you to know where this problem started.

JILL: That feels right. I know that my problem started long before I met my husband. If I see how it started, maybe I could figure out what to do to start being more self-accepting.

THERAPIST: Perhaps you could share some of your memories concerning feelings of not accepting yourself.

Thus, Jill begins to talk about her past difficulties with self-acceptance. In addition to using active listening skills, the therapist may also employ other skills to facilitate patient insight such as interpretations, self-disclosures, and challenges (Hill, 2014).

In contrast to Jill's therapist, Maria's therapist has a cognitive-behavioral theoretical orientation that focuses on changing current thoughts and behaviors by following treatment plans based on behavioral principals. Similar to Jamal's therapist, Maria's therapist is very active in collaborating with her to set up the tasks that Maria will undertake to reach her goal of focusing on what she does well.

MARIA: I like what you just said about focusing on the things I do well rather than on what I screw up. But, I have a hard time telling when I do something well.

THERAPIST: You could keep a diary of relevant events. What things that you do every day or so do you consider important in your life?

MARIA: There are several things I do at work most days that are important.

THERAPIST: You could record each of these things when it happens and then record the outcome of each event.

MARIA: Do you mean to actually write all this down? What if I don't know the outcome?

THERAPIST: Yes, write down the event in as much detail as possible. If you don't know the outcome, don't write anything about outcome. Bring what you write to our next session, and we can discuss each instance.

When Maria returns for her next session, the therapist asks about her feelings concerning each of the recorded instances. Maria was surprised that there were so many instances and was also surprised that her behavior contributed to good outcomes for many of them. They talked about how she can reward herself for contributing to good outcomes at work. Maria decides to record her non-work events as well following the same procedure.

Fred's therapist also has a cognitive-behavioral theoretical orientation. Fred expresses his goal of having a job he enjoys but being afraid that his family will not support his wish.

THERAPIST: It appears that it might easier to pursue a teaching career if you believed that your family would be supportive of whatever you choose.

FRED: It would be so much easier if I had their support.

THERAPIST: Perhaps there is one member of your family whom you believe you could talk to about your dilemma who might support you.

FRED: My older sister has always been in my corner.

THERAPIST: Okay, so how do you feel about role-playing a conversation you might have with your older sister about supporting your career choice? This would allow you to rehearse what you are going to say.

FRED: That might help. I want to explain my situation to her so she will understand it completely because I want to get her support and her help in getting my parent's support.

THERAPIST: You set the scene. Maybe you can first educate me about your sister and how she usually interacts with you. Then I'll role-play her.

Fred and the therapist role-play Fred's recounting his dilemma to his sister and asking for her help. Then they switch roles and the therapist plays Fred, and Fred plays his sister. This allows the therapist to model verbal behaviors that may be the most effective. If, or when, Fred speaks with other family members, he and the therapist can employ similar behavioral rehearsal, modeling, and role-play tasks. But because Fred's goal in part involves trying to modify others' wishes, he may not be able to achieve it.

Jim's therapist has a cognitive-behavioral theoretical orientation and wants to employ behavioral rehearsal and modeling to help Jim have a better relationship with his co-worker and hopefully keep his job. Jim, however, is not particularly enthusiastic about relating to his co-worker in a positive way, nor does he want to role-play.

THERAPIST: What would it look like if you and your co-worker had a better relationship?

JIM: Well, I guess we wouldn't bother each other anymore. I wouldn't speak to him, and he wouldn't speak to me. But, I'm sure that he would manage to get in some little thing and that would set me off. He thinks he can get away with anything.

THERAPIST: Like what?

JIM: Well, he'd say something to someone else about me while I was in earshot or he'd give me a dirty look.

THERAPIST: This doesn't sound like getting along to me.

JIM: It isn't.

THERAPIST: How well do you know him?

JIM: Not well. He hangs out with a group of guys, and they go out together after work.

THERAPIST: Do you know any of these people? Do you know what they do together?

JIM: I know a couple of them, not well, but better than him. I have no idea where they go.

THERAPIST: Perhaps you might approach one of them, see what they do, and ask if you could tag along if you discover that what they do is something that you'd be interested in.

JIM: I suppose I could at least see what they do after work, but I don't want to piss any of them off. Then I'd just be in more trouble.

THERAPIST: We could role-play how you might approach one of them that you know best. Sometimes people find this helpful. You can rehearse what you're going to say.

JIM: I'm not keen on that role-play stuff. I suppose I could just talk to this one guy who doesn't seem so bad.

THERAPIST: What do you think you will say?

JIM: Don't know, just play it by ear.

Although Jim might have a better chance of success if he rehearses the conversation with the therapist, he does not want to do this and the therapist respects his wishes. It is important for therapists to attend to their patients' desires. Otherwise, goal setting is one-sided, patients feel excluded, and they may not follow through with therapy. Throughout the goal-setting process, it is advisable for therapists to seek and incorporate patients' input. This behavior is central to the working alliance.

Assessing Progress Toward Goals

It is essential to monitor patients' goal progress. Progress may be slow or lacking, thus necessitating a change in goals or the tasks to achieve them. Therapists reinforce the importance of attending to goal-related homework tasks by checking on how they are being enacted and, in collaboration with patients, making changes to facilitate their effectiveness. It is important to seek patients' input concerning the "doability" of homework assignments. Thus, Fred's therapist listened to Fred's recounting of his conversation with his sister and provided him with feedback and additional behavioral rehearsal concerning conversations he will next have with other members of his family.

Even if patients have no homework, it is important to begin most sessions by checking on how well patients believe that therapy is going and, in collaboration with patients, make changes to treatment tasks. Asking patients about their progress toward goals also shows therapists' commitment to the treatment process.

In addition to checking homework and obtaining patients' feedback, there are other methods to use for goal progress monitoring. For example, Jamal has a hierarchy of steps to his goal of giving a speech with little anxiety. Jamal rates his anxiety while performing each step on a 10-point scale where 1 represents "no anxiety" and 10 represents "maximal anxiety." He and the therapist can decide when to move to the next step based on his ratings. Each step completed is progress toward his goal.

Idiographic measures of goal attainment are individually customized to patients' needs. One such measure is Goal Attainment Scaling (GAS; Kiresuk & Sherman, 1968), a widely used method of rating goal outcomes. The outcome of each identified goal is rated on a numerical scale, with the points on the scale representing the "least favorable outcome" (−4), the "most likely outcome" (0), and "the most favorable outcome" (+4). The GAS can be used to evaluate several goals at a time. The ratings of each goal can be combined into a single score for an overall goal attainment score. Each of our imaginary patients could use the GAS to appraise his or her goal progress. Although our patients have identified one goal each, many patients have more than one goal, and our imaginary patients may have several goals as well as they continue in treatment. The GAS could be used to assess progress for each of their several goals.

Another idiographic measure of goal progress is the Goal Attainment Form (GAF; Evans et al., 2000). Patients state up to four problems they want to work on at the beginning of therapy. At the end of therapy, patients rate the extent to which therapy was helpful for each problem on a 5-point scale with scores ranging from "not at all helpful" (0) to "extremely helpful" (5). Although GAS and the GAF are used as outcome measures, they may be used during the course of therapy to assess goal progress.

There are also more standard measures to assess goal progress. For instance, Fred is depressed about his career situation. Besides talking to his family about changing his vocation, he may have the additional treatment goal of reducing his depression. The Beck Depression Inventory-II (BDI-II; Beck, Steer, & Brown, 1996) and the Hamilton Depression Rating Scale (HDRS; Hamilton, 1960) are brief standardized measures that Fred and his therapist can use to assess his progress toward being less depressed. Jill also is depressed about the breakup of her marriage. The BDI-II and the HDRS can be used to assess her level of depression. Another popular standardized measure, the Symptom Checklist-90 – Revised (SCL-90-R; Derogatis, 1979) assesses general psychological functioning and may be of benefit to patients who are seeking greater psychological health in general. Similar to idiographic measures, standardized measures can be used throughout therapy to assess progress toward goals.

In many cases, therapists will use several of these instruments in addition to patients' verbal feedback to assess goal progress. Continued monitoring of progress toward patients' goals is essential. If progress is static or declines, therapy tasks, or even goals themselves, may have to be altered. When Jamal had difficulty progressing beyond step 5 of his 11-step public speaking hierarchy, he and his therapist inserted another step before step 6 that was less anxiety provoking and therefore easier to do. After completing this step, Jamal accomplished step 6 without difficulty.

Changing Goals During the Course of Therapy

Sometimes patients want to change goals during therapy. Their life circumstances may change or perhaps they find the work needed to attain their goals to be too difficult and wish to switch to a goal that may be more easily achieved. For instance, Berking et al. (2005) suggest that patients who want to get rid of their sleep problems (the most difficult goal to achieve according to their research) may switch to the more achievable goal of coping with their sleep problems (p. 322).

Similarly, in collaboration with her therapist, imaginary patient Maria switched from her avoidance goal of not being self-critical to a more attainable approach goal of focusing on what she does well. The avoidance goal led to more, instead of less, self-criticism. The approach goal was easier for her to achieve.

Patients also switch goals because they lack the resources they need to attain their goals. For example, imaginary patient Fred wants his parents' support to pursue his goal of becoming a teacher. Although he gained his sister's support in this endeavor, he has been unable to get the backing of his parents, who insist he continue in medical school. Now Fred has a choice to make. Should he stick with his desire to quit medical school and pursue a teaching career, or should he continue in medical school even though he is depressed?

FRED: I'm really discouraged. I thought that with my sister's help we could persuade my parents to support my wish to be a teacher.

THERAPIST: It is very hard to change someone else. We can only change ourselves. How do you see your future if the choice is just up to you?

FRED: I see myself teaching, preferably high school. I really, really, really don't want to be a doctor, but I don't want to hurt my parents either.

This interchange is the beginning of a collaborative discussion to allow Fred to choose to pursue his goal of being a teacher without his parents' support. The tasks to reach his goal include insight into his relationship with his parents and cognitive restructuring to challenge his automatic thoughts about his value as a son.

Discussing Termination from a Goal Perspective

At the beginning of this chapter, I indicated that it is not unusual for patient and therapist to meet regularly with little determination of what the desired endpoint might be. This situation makes it almost impossible to tell what constitutes patient improvement. Directionless, open-ended therapy can sometimes go on for years, with patients feeling as if they are "drifting along through life getting from day to day—surviving but not living" (Feltham et al., p. 74). It is also possible for patients to go on for years and to say continually that they feel better, feel supported, and value their therapy and therapist, but still it may be difficult to ascertain what constitutes improvement.

Regardless of the theoretical orientation of the therapist, therapy from a goal perspective provides a desired endpoint—achievement of patients' goals. Collaborative goal-setting establishes agreed-upon goals and the methods to reach them. It also allows for assessment of progress toward goals. This does not mean that all goals are reached at therapy termination. Indeed, many terminations occur because of situations other than goal achievement. Patients or therapists may move away from the area and thus not be able to continue treatment with each other. Patients' insurance may permit fewer sessions than needed. The agency where the therapy takes place may have duration limits.

Patients may also believe that it is not necessary to totally achieve their goals; improvement in their problems may be sufficient. Law (2018) advocates talking about therapy's ending from the very beginning of treatment. He suggests telling patients that they can work with the therapist for as long as it is helpful. Thus, even though the goal is not completely or perfectly achieved, if patients are satisfied with where they currently are in the goal process or believe that they are far enough along to continue progressing by themselves, therapy termination can take place. By monitoring and discussing goal progress throughout therapy, patients and therapist can anticipate when it will end.

Our imaginary patients terminated under various circumstances. Jamal and Maria both reached their treatment goals. Jamal gave his classroom speech with minimal anxiety, received an A– for the speech, and got a B+ for the course grade. Maria rated herself as having a greater focus on what she does well at termination and expressed a continuing desire to look at the positives, rather than the negatives, in her life. Jill gained considerable insight into the origins of her problem with self-acceptance. She terminated believing that she could now make decisions that benefitted her rather than relying on others. Fred continued treatment until the end of the semester, when he could no longer see the therapist provided by the medical school. Both he and his therapist believed that he needed further treatment to achieve his goals, so he accepted a referral to a low-cost clinic. He got a job teaching science at a private school and is working to save enough money to return to school to get a teaching certificate. Although he feels somewhat less guilty about disappointing his parents, he needs further help with this issue. Jim did not try to talk to his co-worker and continued to tease him at work. He left therapy after four sessions and was ultimately fired from his job.

Besides collaborating with patients concerning goal progress, therapists have other tasks to perform to ensure a smooth termination. Termination research (summarized by Gelso & Woodhouse, 2002) indicates that, in addition to setting a termination date and reviewing goal attainment, therapists discuss plans for the future with their patients. This discussion often includes an invitation to return to treatment if the need arises as well as a referral for additional help if necessary. Therapists also address closure in the therapist–patient relationship. Patient and therapist discuss their feelings about ending the relationship, and both parties may share feelings about the therapy process. Patients may ask therapists personal questions, and patient and therapist relate to each other as equals. Many patients seek treatment off and on during their lives. It is important to ensure a positive treatment ending even when not all goals were realized and the working alliance between therapist and patient may not have been ideal. A frank discussion of what transpired during the course of therapy underscores the notion that therapists believe that it is important for patients' voices to be heard. This belief may facilitate patients' seeking additional therapy when needed.

Summary

Therapist–patient agreement on the goals and tasks of psychotherapy is a key ingredient of the working alliance. Collaborative goal setting gives therapy direction, allows for assessment of progress, and provides an endpoint. This chapter presents therapists with methods to achieve goal consensus with patients, beginning with the use of active listening skills to assess patients' problems and determine what goals patients and therapists will address. Goal choices are made in patients' best interest, and therapists and patients reformulate goals that are unsafe or will be difficult to achieve to safer, more easily achieved goals. Next, patients and therapists collaboratively determine the tasks that will facilitate achievement of the patients' goal. Therapy tasks are influenced by the therapist's theoretical orientation in conjunction with input from the patients. It is important to regularly assess goal progress and to routinely seek patients' input. Therapy tasks, or even goals themselves, may need modification if they prove too difficult to effect. Termination occurs when goals are fully or almost fully achieved.

References

Beck, A. T., Steer, R. A., & Brown, G. K. (1996). *Beck Depression Inventory—II*. San Antonio, TX: Psychological Corporation.

Berking, M., Grosse Holtforth, M., Jacobi, C., & Kröner-Herwig, B. (2005). Empirically based goal-finding procedures in psychotherapy: Are some goals easier to attain than others? *Psychotherapy Research, 15*, 316–324. doi:10.1080/10503300500091801

Bordin, E. S. (1979). The generalizability of the psychoanalytic concept of the working alliance. *Psychotherapy Theory, Research, Practice, Training, 16*, 252–260. doi:10.1037/h0085885

Cooper, M. (2018). The psychology of goals: A practice-friendly review. In M. Cooper & D. Law (Eds.), *Working with goals in psychotherapy and counselling* (pp. 35–71). Oxford: Oxford University Press.

Derogatis, L. R. (1979). *Symptom Checklist-90-Revised (SCL-90-R)*. Lyndhurst, NJ: NCS Pearson.

Elliot, A. J., & Church, M. A. (2002). Client-articulated avoidance goals in the therapy context. *Journal of Counseling Psychology, 49*, 243–254. doi:10.1037/0022-0167.49.2.243

Evans, C., Mellor-Clark, J., Margison, F., Barkham, M., Audin, K., Connell, J., ... McGrath, G. (2000). CORE: Clinical Outcomes in Routine Evaluation. *Journal of Mental Health, 9*, 247–255. doi:1080/jmh.9.3.247.255

Feltham, A., Martin, K., Walker, L., & Harris, L. (2018). Using goals in therapy: The perspective of people with lived experience. In M. Cooper & D. Law (Eds.), *Working with goals in psychotherapy and counselling* (pp. 73–86). Oxford: Oxford University Press.

Gelso, C. J., & Woodhouse, S. S. (2002). The termination of psychotherapy: What research tells us about the process of ending treatment. In G. S. Tryon (Ed.), *Counseling based on process research: Applying what we know* (pp. 344–369). Boston: Allyn and Bacon.

Hamilton, M. A. (1960). A rating scale for depression. *Journal of Neurology, Neurosurgery and Psychiatry, 23*, 56–62.

Hill, C. E. (2014). *Helping skills: Facilitating exploration, insight, and action* (4th ed.). Washington, DC: American Psychological Association.

Kiresuk, T. J., & Sherman, M. R. E. (1968). Goal attainment scaling: A general method for evaluating comprehensive community mental health programs. *Community Mental Health Journal, 4,* 443–453. doi:10.1007/BF01530764

Law, D. (2018). Goal-oriented practice. In M. Cooper and D. Law (Eds.), *Working with goals in psychotherapy and counselling* (pp. 161–180). Oxford: Oxford University Press.

Michalak, J., & Grosse Holtforth, M. (2006). Where do we go from here? The goal perspective in psychotherapy. *Clinical Psychology: Science and Practice, 13,* 346–365. doi:10.1111/j.1468-2850.2006.00048.x

Rogers, C. R. (1957). The necessary and sufficient conditions of therapeutic personality change. *Journal of Consulting Psychology, 21,* 95–103. doi.org/10.1037/h0045357

Swift, J., & Callahan, J. (2009). Early psychotherapy processes: An examination of client and trainee clinician perspective convergence. *Clinical Psychology and Psychotherapy, 16,* 228–236. doi:10.1002/cpp.617

Tryon, G. S., Birch, S. E., & Verkuilen, J. (2018). Meta-analyses of the relation of goal consensus and collaboration to psychotherapy outcome. *Psychotherapy, 55.* doi:10.1037/pst0000170

Zane, N., Sue, S., Chang, J., Huang, L., Huang, J., Lowe, S. . . . Lee, E. (2005). Beyond ethnic match: Effects of client-therapist cognitive match in problem perception, coping orientation, and therapy goals on treatment outcomes. *Journal of Community Psychology, 33,* 569–585. doi:10.1002/jcop.20067

5

Consensus and Collaboration in the Working Alliance

Jairo N. Fuertes, Michael T. Moore, and Chloe C. Pagano-Stalzer

While the working alliance was operationalized by Bordin (1979) in terms of the level of agreement between therapist and client on the goals and tasks of therapy and as an emotional bond characterized by trust between the two, the working alliance goes beyond this operational definition and is more precisely characterized by a sense of consensus, collaboration, and shared mission that exists between therapist and client (Gelso, 2006; Hatcher & Barends, 2006). In discussing the relationship between Bordin's goals, tasks, and bond, and the broader constructs of consensus and collaboration inherent in the working alliance, Gelso and Hayes (1998) theorized that they are highly related and that they "influence and are influenced by" each other. That is, agreement on goals and tasks and the emotional bond that exists between the therapist and client influence and are influenced by the level of consensus and collaboration between the participants. In this chapter, we focus on how therapists can go about developing and maintaining a sense of consensus and collaboration with clients. We also present what we have identified as "markers" of consensus and collaboration in therapy: collaborative motivation, framework consensus, and collaborative action.

What does it mean to be "allies"? The *Oxford English Dictionary* tells us that allies unite or connect in a formal or close relationship or bond. Clinically speaking, to us it means the momentary meeting or joining together of the participants' minds/psyches to solve specific problems or to try to uncover, identify, and/or resolve problems for the client. This sense of being together may or may not involve setting goals and/or identifying tasks to meet the goals, but it certainly means the establishment of a professional relationship where at least some level of consensus, collaboration, and trust is essential. An alliance can exist in a relationship where goals are rarely if ever discussed, but it cannot exist, in our view, in a relationship where the participants do not share a sense of being on a common venture or mission. Reaching a working alliance characterized by a sense of consensus and collaboration inevitably requires conscious and deliberate practice on the part of the therapist. This is important, given evidence that shows that some clients see their therapy in general, and the working alliance in particular, differently from the way that their therapists sees them (Bedi, Davis, & Arvay, 2005); there is also evidence that clients' views of the alliance are generally better associated with outcome (Flückiger, Del Re, Wampold, & Horvath, 2018). Deliberate practice on the part of the therapist is also warranted given the evidence that the working alliance is different for each client; that is, the working alliance is co-created between a therapist and a client, and it takes on the qualities and contributions made by each of the participants (Chapter 6).

Consensus and Collaboration

Consensus is defined by Merriam-Webster as "general agreement about something, an idea or opinion that is shared by people in a group." In therapy, consensus means to us that there is a general agreement between the therapist and the client about specific ideas, observations, feelings, etc., and/or the general content of the discussion taking place. It means that both the therapist and client feel that they see eye-to-eye, so to speak, about what is being discussed, planned, or evaluated. Consensus appears to be key to the therapist and client developing some type of collaboration and to developing a sense of being allies in a shared mission in the work. Consistent with Gelso and Hayes (1998), we see consensus and collaboration as influencing and being influenced by Bordin's agreement on tasks and goals, as well as by the experience of trust between therapist and client. However, consensus and collaboration can be evident even in the absence of specified goals or tasks. For example, there can be consensus between participants in therapies where goals and tasks are not necessarily discussed or specified. While the focus of this chapter could be exclusively on the importance of achieving and maintaining consensus in treatment, we see much of the working alliance as also involving collaboration, and the latter depends, in our view, on some level of consensus having been established.

Wikipedia defines *collaboration* as "the process of two or more people or organizations working together to complete a task or achieve a goal." In our view, there can be consensus without collaboration, for example when participants agree about the nature and severity of a problem but the client has not decided whether he or she is ready to work on the problem. But it seems unfathomable to us to see two people collaborating in therapy without some measure of agreement on the nature of a problem or about the course of action. In the remainder of this chapter, we discuss consensus *and* collaboration, since they are closely related phenomena, and see, at the heart of the matter, the importance of the therapist and client sharing in the complexity of what the client discusses and, to some extent, the two agreeing on the problems and possible solutions to whatever concerns the client has. Just as Bordin conceptualized the alliance as a pan-theoretical phenomenon evident in all therapies, we see consensus and collaboration as evident in all forms of psychotherapy. While there are more than 30 measures of the alliance in the literature (Horvath, Del Re, Flückiger, & Symonds, 2011), the vast majority of the research has used the following four measures: the California Psychotherapy Alliance Scale (CALPAS; Gaston & Marmar, 1994), the Helping Alliance Questionnaires (HAQ; Alexander & Luborsky, 1987), the Vanderbilt Psychotherapy Process Scale (VPPS; O'Mally, Suh, & Strupp, 1983), and the Working Alliance Inventory (WAI; Horvath & Greenberg, 1986; Horvath et al., 2011). As Horvath et al. (2011) reported, a factor analysis of these four measures has yielded a "central common theme" (p. 28) among them, referred to as a "confident collaborative relationship" by Hatcher and Barends (1996). Our discussion here focuses on clinical practice and ways in which therapists can go about fostering a "confident collaborative relationship."

Approaches to Consensus and Collaboration

Consensus and collaboration can be fostered by an array of interventions available to therapists, and these stem from therapists' theoretical and technical approaches to treatment. Just as Bordin's definition of the working alliance was intended to be pan-theoretical (i.e., not explicitly tied to one particular therapeutic orientation or another), we see consensus and collaboration as essential to and evident in all forms of therapy. Therapists working from a variety of perspectives/traditions strive to get the client to engage as fully as possible in the work of treatment. Psychoanalytic/dynamic therapists may convey to their clients that they seek to understand the client as deeply and completely as possible; they may emphasize, for example, understanding the client's defenses, wishes, fantasies, personal history, etc. In order for that to take place, the client has to open up and share as much as possible about him- or herself. The humanist/existential therapist will work to connect with the client in a meaningful, authentic, and safe way and will try to understand the client's perspective as closely as possible as the client sees and feels it, so that the client can be more fully and authentically present. Therapists operating from a cognitive-behavioral approach will work to understand and identify a concrete problem that is vexing for the client and then develop/tailor a workable and doable plan (with possibly several steps or stages) that fits with the client in order to make changes in thoughts, feelings, and behaviors.

There are several commonalities across the different schools of psychotherapy. For example, all therapists are trained to listen deeply and carefully, in a way that is usually not done in other relationships. Generally, clients talk and therapists listen. The skills associated with active deep listening include the therapist clearing his or her mind to the extent possible for the client, putting personal concerns aside to be able to respond to the client, making engaging eye contact with the client, focusing, and nodding appropriately as the client talks. Clinical wisdom suggests that a good rule of thumb is for the client to speak about 75% of the session, and, while there are substantial differences evident in therapist talk time between therapies, this percentage is generally reflective of our clinical experience. Also, therapists tend to think about cases between sessions and come prepared to work during the sessions (albeit, with an open mind and being receptive to new material). Therapists strive to understand how their clients view and experience their problems. The skills associated with deep listening are many but include empathy and various types of probes. Clinical practice generally involves listening, the use of empathy, and developing tentative hypotheses about the nature of the problems that the client experiences using the material generated by probes. Therapists generally prioritize the problems that they believe require the most immediate attention and, finally, share clinically indicated aspects of their thinking with their clients.

To establish *consensus*, we generally share how we see the problem and check continuously with the client to see if it fits with how they see the problem. We ask our clients whether they agree with our conceptualization of their problem, and we ask for feedback and input to get the clearest possible picture of what the client is thinking and experiencing. We clarify roles by noting that while we care for and are working for our clients, they are ultimately responsible for making all decisions related to their lives. We also communicate "rules" for the treatment, including the length of sessions, limits to confidentiality, communications between sessions, and the like. This is all part of establishing parameters of honesty, trust, and respect and contribute to developing a "just society" (Egan, 2010) in the relationship, one "based on mutual respect and planning" (p. 123).

We also communicate the importance of honesty and trust, and, to varying degrees, we convey the importance of being on the same page, as the saying goes. It is important to note that we actively *invite collaboration*. We share with the client that therapy is a collaborative process, and, in this way, we try to develop a spirit of consensus in the work, a sense of mutuality, and/or the belief that the treatment is a shared mission. It seems reasonable to assume that clients have some notion of needing to do something about their problem(s); that is why they came to therapy (unless, of course, they were mandated to enter therapy, and even then, clients may have some idea that they have a problem). We see our task as therapists to deliberately tap and foster that spirit of collaboration with the client, so that he or she can, in turn, collaborate with us as therapists. Questions that foster this spirit of collaboration include "How does this sound to you?" "Do you agree or disagree with this?" "What do you think?" "What do you propose?"

"Does it make sense to you?" "Does this sound like something that would be helpful to you?" We use "we" and "us" statements that foster that sense of being together in the work.

Since the purpose of this volume is to enhance clinical practice with respect to the working alliance, we present several case examples that can help to demonstrate these concepts. As the reader will note, there is a decidedly cognitive-behavioral flavor to many of the clinical examples presented and discussed here; this is because we tend to intervene by focusing on clients' cognitions and behaviors. While this may be the predominating approach in the examples that follow, there are many approaches to achieving consensus and collaboration on the basis of personal theory and technique.

Consensus and Collaboration from the Beginning to the End of Therapy

In our estimation, the sense of being allies is crucial at the beginning stages of therapy as it gives the client hope and it encourages exploration and the initial steps toward change. The first few sessions of therapy are often focused on assessment. In this stage, the therapist gets to know the client (and vice versa), and the focus and/or the goals and tasks for therapy are established and agreed on. Clients may be hesitant at first to divulge things about themselves, especially events or aspects of themselves associated with guilt or shame. Establishing a sense of being on the same page with the therapist can help the client open up and disclose information that may be essential to understanding the client more fully or completely. The available research on the role of goal consensus and collaboration supports this notion, and these two elements have been deemed "demonstrably effective" (see Norcross & Wampold, 2011, for a review). The Task Force on Evidence-Based Therapy Relationships, in reviewing the available literature, made four recommendations related to practice (Norcross & Wampold, 2011; Norcross & Lambert, 2018). One of these relates directly to consensus and collaboration and states that "Practitioners are encouraged to routinely monitor patients' responses to the therapy relationship and ongoing treatment. Such monitoring leads to increased opportunities to reestablish collaboration, improve the relationship, modify technical strategies, and avoid premature termination" (p. 424). This statement, in addition to emphasizing the importance of collaboration in psychotherapy, also makes the important point that collaboration is an *ongoing process* in psychotherapy and requires routine monitoring. Some researchers and clinicians may think about agreement on the goals and tasks of therapy as a one-time event, to be checked off as a to-do list in the first few sessions and then mostly ignored for the duration of therapy. In actuality, the goals and tasks of therapy may change as client motivation changes and as clients' understanding of both themselves and the process of psychotherapy develops.

In the middle stages of therapy, the sense of being allies helps in challenging clients and in dealing with strains or ruptures in the alliance, perhaps when the client fully grasps the complexity of the problem or when she or he starts making changes that are difficult, painful, and/or scary. After the initial development of a case conceptualization (the case conceptualization process should *also* be ongoing) and alliance development, therapy can enter a middle phase in which intervention becomes more prominent and assessment less so. The intensity or frequency of some interventions may change. For example, a therapist may start offering more interpretations, revealing possibilities and connections that go beyond the client's direct experience, or a therapist may engage in exposure exercises that gradually become more challenging. Cognitive work progresses from a focus on immediate thoughts to a focus on core beliefs that underlie these thoughts. Regardless of the school of psychotherapy, the work of therapy can become more difficult in the middle phase of therapy, and a sustained sense of consensus and collaboration may be essential for the client to feel that he or she has a partner in the increasingly difficult work that is being done and that the work is for the client's benefit. A sense of having a partner in the therapist can encourage and help justify the discomfort the client may increasingly feel in the middle stages of therapy. In addition to the research reviewed earlier on the benefits of collaboration, the Task Force on Evidence-Based Therapy Relationships (Norcross & Wampold, 2011) also reviewed evidence that supported the notion that the *lack* of collaboration is harmful in psychotherapy and stated that "Paucity of empathy, collaboration, consensus, and positive regard predict treatment dropout and failure" (p. 427).

In the latter stages of therapy, a continued sense of consensus and collaboration can help clients continue toward action, solidify changes, and gain greater confidence in their ability to cope and their ability to develop other allies and supports after therapy ends. At the end of therapy, clients venture out into the world without the emotional safety of the working alliance. Still, if therapy has gone well, the working alliance has been, to one degree or another, taken inside or internalized. In addition, the renewed sense of independence brings its own stresses and challenges; for example, how to prevent relapses and/or the challenge of how to cope with symptoms and situations without the benefit of the therapist.

Fostering Consensus and Collaboration

It is our opinion that therapists can communicate intentionally and deliberately in a manner that develops and maintains consensus and collaboration in therapy. The goal for most therapists is to help clients to think, feel, and behave in ways that are healthier and more adaptive. With clients who have *persistent and/or significant* problems, ambivalence can be the rule rather than the exception in psychotherapy, to adopt the language and the thinking in Motivational Interviewing (Miller & Rollnick, 2012). Therefore, the question that will guide our discussion of the techniques that we believe foster consensus and collaboration is: "How do you engage your client in the work of therapy?" A deliberate approach can help therapists foster consensus and collaboration, much in the same way that deliberate practice can enhance treatment outcomes in therapy (Chow et al., 2015; Goldberg et al., 2016).

Client collaboration has been discussed as a primary factor in the process and outcome of therapy (Lambert, 1992; Orlinsky, Rønnestad, & Willutzki, 2004), and the most recent meta-analysis on this topic has provided support for this notion. Tryon, Birch, and Verkuilen (2018) provided evidence of a medium effect of the relationship between therapist–client collaboration and outcome in therapy ($r = .29$, or $d = .61$). However, the limitations of the current research on collaboration make it impossible to distinguish between unique client and therapist contributions (Tryon et al., 2018). There is also some medical literature connecting patient activation (i.e., conceptualized as increased motivation, knowledge, skills, and confidence to manage one's health) with general health and management of chronic health conditions (e.g., Greene, Hibbard, Sacks, Overton, & Parrotta, 2015; Hibbard, Mahoney, Stock, & Tusler, 2007; O'Malley, Dewan, Ohman-Strickland, Gundersen, Miller, & Hudson, 2018). In both the psychotherapy and the medical literatures, client/patient collaboration has mostly been measured using concrete criteria, such as homework compliance or medication or diet compliance. While these are viable markers of patient collaboration, from our theoretical and clinical perspectives, there are three markers of client behavior that signal consensus and collaboration, and we want to note these in this chapter (please note that Bedi and Hayes in Chapter 6 of this volume discuss client factors in-depth). The client is key to the success of therapy, and without his or her input, collaboration, and hard work, even the best therapist would have very limited outcomes. Clients should feel like active participants in the therapy; that therapy is being done *with* them, not *to* them. When consensus and collaboration are fostered by the therapist, they tend to activate clients with a sense of being important team members in the therapy and that they share at times being in the driver's seat, with significant say and influence in their treatment.

Collaborative Motivation

In our clinical experience there are three interrelated markers of client behavior that signal that there is consensus and collaboration in the dyad: collaborative motivation, framework consensus, and collaborative action. These three phenomena are interrelated (i.e., we predict that they share considerable variance), are evident throughout therapy, and each influences and is influenced by the others. Collaborative motivation goes beyond what the client brings in terms of motivation at the beginning of treatment; collaborative motivation refers to the client becoming motivated with the therapist as therapy progresses, it is a motivation that involves the therapist as an ally and is there throughout the course of treatment. If the therapist is a guide and/or companion on a healing journey, then collaborative motivation is when the two, therapist and client, become allies in a journey that they will take together, even before they know where the journey is heading or how they are going to get there. Attending to collaborative motivation is important because a client who is initially highly motivated to do the work of therapy may find that this motivation drops when the difficult work of therapy begins. Without the therapist deliberately attending to dips or fluctuations in client motivation and discussing it explicitly as an ally, the progress of therapy may be negatively affected.

The following example demonstrates how collaborative motivation over the course of therapy can help.

Virginia, 51, came to therapy to help her cope with the sudden and unexpected loss of her 19-year-old son. She was married and had two other children: her oldest son had recently moved out of state for graduate school, and her youngest daughter had recently begun attending college at a local university. At intake, she described feeling depressed, being almost completely unable to experience pleasure from anything, feeling intensely (and unreasonably) guilty and responsible for her son's death, and feeling as though she lost a majority of her sense of purpose with two of three children no longer in her care. She was initially highly motivated to participate in therapy, enjoyed the individual attention and the catharsis, and attended regularly. However, over time, the focus of sessions shifted from identifying her thoughts and feelings to probing them more deeply. The topic of the sessions progressed into the meaning of the loss and the context in which it occurred, including problems she had in her relationships with her remaining family members. Virginia found understanding her feelings and talking about her fraught relationships much less rewarding than the venting that characterized earlier sessions. Her attendance began to dip, and she seemed less active and involved in session. The therapist talked to her about what she wanted to get out of their sessions together and how just venting would not allow her to achieve her long-terms goals for therapy. They discussed that, while venting felt good in the moment, it would not teach her how to cope with the feelings for which she had expressed wanting help. The therapist recognized how difficult the work would be but emphasized the long-term benefits, how doing the work would allow her to enjoy activities she valued, and that they would be going through the process together. After a discussion, Virginia responded with general agreement; she came to see that she had been too focused on how good venting felt and that expressing, but not understanding or processing her thoughts and feelings, was not consistent with what she wanted to accomplish in therapy, over the long term. Therapy progressed with a renewed energy on Virginia's part; she was more actively engaged in session, and her attendance improved. There was still hard work to do, but she was motivated to do it and felt a renewed connection with her therapist.

The case of Virginia illustrates how motivation can change as therapy progresses and how collaboration can help motivate the client toward the difficult work in treatment. Clients can become ambivalent or even resistant about the work in treatment for a variety of reasons, and this ambivalence needs to be openly discussed in order to regain a sense of shared purpose and direction in treatment.

A question that therapists could ask themselves when trying to initiate change with their client is if the change is linked to the client's beliefs or values. Is it clear how the change will allow the client to engage in a valued role (or reach for or work for a valued goal)? For example, is it valuable or meaningful to the client to be a better parent/spouse/friend/employee/student? If this is not immediately obvious, it is worth exploring this with the client. Second, it should be clear how the change is both connected to one or more of the client's stated goals for therapy (whether the goals are specific or broad) and *essential* for the goal(s) to be realized. The following example illustrates these points where the issue of homework is being introduced.

Liam, 48, is seeking therapy for his long-standing feelings of depression and pessimism, both of which have been issues "for as long as I can remember." The therapist, to assist in both the formation of a case conceptualization and for the purpose of outcomes assessment, has decided to offer a self-monitoring homework assignment involving recording the duration and intensity of feelings of sadness and pessimistic and self-defeating thoughts, as well as the content of these thoughts. The therapist described the assignment in the last 5 minutes of the session and asked Liam to complete it. The following week, Liam reported that he only completed the assignment on 2 days. Upon reflection and consultation with a colleague, the therapist realized that he assumed that Liam would understand why the homework was important because the link to his presenting problems seemed "obvious." The therapist assumed that Liam would be motivated to do the homework because it would help reduce his symptoms. In the next session, the therapist opened with an exploration of what changes in himself Liam wanted to see from therapy, to ensure that both Liam and the therapist were on the same page. Liam said that he wanted to reduce his feelings of sadness and wanted to have a better opinion of himself and, especially, of others. However, Liam also admitted to feeling ambivalent about reducing his symptoms. "To be honest doc, I'm not really sure who I am, other than being 'the sad guy.'" The therapist talked with Liam about his ambivalence about reducing his symptoms and who he was, outside of his sadness. The therapist also attempted to link the homework assignment to Liam's values and explained that it would help him to develop an idea for how his feelings of sadness were linked to his pessimistic and self-defeating thoughts and other events in Liam's life. Specifically, the therapist stated that recording the frequency of his sad feelings would help the therapist to know whether the interventions implemented in therapy were working. He also explained how this was particularly important in people suffering from depression, as they have a tendency to perceive their achievements to be less significant than they are, including progress in therapy. Without knowing what caused his sadness, there was no way to know how to reduce it, and without assessing his sadness, there was no way to know whether he was getting better or worse. Liam responded that he understood and committed to completing the homework. The following week, he completed his self-monitoring homework every day.

In this example, the therapist made the mistake of assuming that Liam was motivated to reduce his sadness and assigning homework without linking the assignment to one of Liam's goals for treatment (i.e., what he wanted and valued). Liam was ambivalent about symptom improvement. He was unsure how completing the homework would help him feel less sad and pessimistic and improve his opinions of himself or others, and therefore he did not complete the homework as assigned. The therapist was able to help Liam work through his ambivalence and link completing the homework to therapeutic improvement that Liam valued, and this had the effect of helping him to feel like an active participant in his own recovery.

As mentioned earlier, an important aspect in establishing consensus and collaboration is understanding the different roles that the client has and the value involved in these roles. Clients' goals are linked to some extent to what they value, and these values are also linked to their roles in life. For example, the client in substance abuse counseling may be motivated by goals linked to his or her roles as parent, spouse, or employee, and the process of maintaining sobriety may be differently linked to these roles. For example, if the client in substance abuse counseling is involved with a romantic partner who encourages substance misuse, valuing this relationship may create tension and ambivalence. The extent to which there is collaborative motivation, consensus on the frame for therapy, and action may very well entail recognition that the client's problems are likely embedded in and should be viewed from the lenses of multiple relationships. These relationships include the client in relation to him- or herself, the client in relation to the therapist and other clients, as significant other/spouse, parent, as member of an extended family, and as co-worker, friend, and member of a community, just to name a few. In certain therapies or with certain clients, it can be valuable to include significant others in the treatment. The following case exemplifies this point.

Jacob, 46, lived with his wife, Carol, and two children and came to therapy because his drinking was causing problems in his work and making it difficult for him to be an effective parent. The therapist had suggested that Jacob try to avoid people, places, and things that had been closely tied to his drinking, and Jacob agreed that this was a good idea. However, week after week, Jacob admitted that he was still going to one bar that he frequented, where he would inevitably see his old friends who pressured him to drink. He would typically give in to this continued pressure. He admitted that while he didn't want to go to the bar, he felt motivated by a desire to carry out the goal he had agreed to in therapy and a desire to satisfy his wife's request that he become a more attentive parent. He started making efforts to be more involved with his kids, and one way to do so was by transporting his children to and from karate class, which was located in the same strip mall as his favorite bar. Jacob felt that refusing to bring his children to karate would be viewed by his wife as another instance of his lack of interest in contributing to the parenting of his two children. Carol was invited to the session and provided with psychoeducation on alcoholism and its treatment. The therapist explained how the strip mall and the bar presented Jacob with cues to drinking and how avoidance of these cues, particularly at the beginning of treatment, would help Jacob to establish a period of sobriety. Carol replied that she understood and suggested other ways that Jacob could contribute to parenting the children so that he no longer felt guilty for not taking them to karate. By the end of the session, both Carol and Jacob reported feeling a bit closer and of having a better sense of them being united in helping Jacob in his sobriety. Jacob said that he felt renewed hope in "tackling *our* problem, instead of *my* problem."

In this example, the therapist recognized that a key barrier to Jacob's success was the incompatibility of his desire to avoid cues to drink with his desire to take his children to karate class. The therapist also recognized that resolving this incompatibility with Jacob's wife would be far easier than attempting to resolve it in her absence and that there would be value in marshalling Jacob's resources in his close relationships. The therapist was able to develop consensus with Jacob on the nature of his problem and on the powerful role his wife, Carol, played in motivating him toward sobriety. Making progress on the goal required that Jacob was in agreement with the therapist that (1) his values were in conflict, (2) this conflict frustrated his attempts at sobriety, and (3) his wife had an important role to play in resolving this conflict of values. Consensus and collaboration in this case involved Jacob and the therapist, as well as Jacob and his wife. Once everyone was on the same page, therapy could move forward again.

Framework Consensus

In building and maintaining a collaborative atmosphere in therapy, it is important that both the therapist and client be on the same page about the general parameters/boundaries of the work and about the nuts and bolts of the treatment if these latter have been or are to be specified. Consensus on the frame involves having a sense of agreement about the direction and pace of therapy, and also possibly its duration. Framework consensus is broader than just agreement on the goals and tasks of treatment; it implies that the therapist and client share a high level of mutuality about the mission of counseling, even if that mission is altered or changes in objective with the progression of therapy. Framework consensus is closely related to collaborative motivation, and each influences the other.

As mentioned earlier in the chapter, in our view, consensus and collaboration do not only refer to the goals and tasks of therapy. Both are both possible and vitally important before goals and tasks are defined and at those times in therapy when no specific goals for therapy are articulated. This is also the case for consensus with regard to knowledge: it is beneficial for the work of therapy that therapist and client to agree on shared values of therapy even when these values do not constitute a goal for that therapy. The following example illustrates this point.

Henry, 68, came to therapy after years of suffering with a painful autoimmune disorder that required frequent hospitalizations for treatment. He had worked as a therapist himself for several decades and reported to the therapist that he didn't want any therapy that was going to focus on changing his thoughts or his behavior. "I don't blame myself or have any overly negative beliefs about my illness. I don't need advice, I've heard it all." Brief conversation confirmed that this was true. Henry's thoughts and behaviors were just fine, but the reality of his situation caused him to feel reasonably frustrated, and he wanted help with that. Instead of focusing on his negative feelings and his various pains, and trying to reduce Henry's suffering and help him solve his problems, the therapist tried a different tack. The therapist replied: "I hear what you're saying, Henry. You've had a lifetime of experience with helping people cope and I doubt I could add to how you've already tried to reframe your own experience. What I think I might be able to do, if this sounds okay to you, is just sit and listen. I'd bet that the load you're carrying, and it's a considerable weight, would seem a lot lighter, and your journey through your illness a lot shorter, if you had someone to share it with. Someone, perhaps, who can appreciate the uniquely difficult place that you're in as a helper who is in the position of having to ask for help. What do you think?" Henry replied in agreement that he would appreciate having someone to listen; a relationship where he didn't have to worry about how the other person would react to his troubles or if he was dominating too much of the conversation.

In this example, it wasn't entirely clear what the goal of the therapy was. Henry was looking for help in dealing with the reality of his illness, but it would be a mistake to say that the goal was to help him with "coping," and Henry would likely bristle at any attempt to teach him coping skills. He needed to connect with another person and needed company on his journey. By coming to an understanding and accepting what Henry's needs and values were and about the parameters that would guide the therapy, the therapist helped Henry to feel heard and understood and laid the necessary groundwork for the work of therapy to commence.

Collaborative Action

The final marker of consensus and collaboration is whether or not after one or, more likely, several sessions of psychotherapy the client is ready to move forward. Action can involve a specific goals (e.g., a 28-year-old professional with a good job who has been contemplating finally moving out of her parent's house and is now ready to look for her own apartment), or action can mean just moving forward in life (e.g., a 51-year-old man who has been grieving the death of his spouse for 2 years).

Collaborative action can include small steps, including the first attempts at engaging in tasks to meet some goal(s) in therapy, or it can include more complex, challenging steps that help reach and even transcend the original goals set in counseling. When we think in therapy of action, we often think that it resides strongly with the client, but our use of the term "collaborative" indicates that the therapist is in fact working closely with the client in the process. The therapist is there with the client, providing support, feedback, monitoring, and evaluating the next set of steps. Working from our cognitive-behavioral perspective, the process of collaborative action involves the process of skill building and taking progressive steps toward some possible goal or outcome. The focus on action is intended to emphasize how skill building can involve both smaller action steps, progressive iterations and gradual shaping of a desired behavior, or larger therapeutic gains that can transcend the client's own identified goals for the therapy. The importance of clients having the knowledge and skills to engage in the work in treatment and, importantly, to be prepared emotionally for the next phase of the work, is illustrated in the following example.

Patricia, 21, was a marketing major at a local university. She was a hard worker who had always achieved above-average grades until recently. Her classwork increasingly involved giving presentations to her classmates in the form of marketing pitches. She was always highly anxious when having to present in class but had also managed to avoid having to do it (usually by self-disclosing her anxiety and asking for an alternative assignment) until now. Her professors increasingly informed her that learning how to present her work in front of co-workers was both an integral part of the work in the field and that pitches were an essential and unavoidable part of classwork. At intake, she expressed feeling defeated by these negative experiences and hopeless that she could ever catch up to the skill level of her classmates with regard to public speaking. This hopelessness was evident in session in Patricia's reluctance to engage with the therapist and complete homework assignments. The therapist discussed how therapy would involve public speaking assignments that would gradually increase in difficulty, beginning with making a pitch to the therapist only and moving up to pitching marketing ideas to strangers who were coached to be more deliberately antagonistic. The therapist predicted that, in the first few exercises, Patricia would learn that it was possible to manage her anxiety, a fact that was less obvious when the stakes were higher and her anxiety was elevated to the level of a panic attack. Success in these early exercises would break the cycle of defeat resulting in hopelessness and decreased effort to improve her public speaking skills. Patricia responded that beginning with making a pitch to the therapist seemed reasonable and, while difficult, was something that she could do. After a few pitches to the therapist, the therapist repeated this conversation to make sure that Patricia continued to feel that what she was being asked to do in therapy was within her abilities. This time, Patricia replied that, given how well the first few pitches went, she actually wanted to accelerate the schedule that had been discussed previously and move directly to pitches to a group of 20 strangers (closely mimicking her classroom experiences). She added that continuing to do one-on-one pitches to the therapist was becoming boring as she felt that she had learned everything she could about managing her mild anxiety in this situation.

In this case example, the therapist and client arrived at a consensus about the goals and tasks of treatment *and* ensured that Patricia was motivated at the outset of therapy. Then, once therapy had started, the therapist returned to this topic to check in, giving Patricia the opportunity to offer that she would prefer to increase the difficulty of the practice pitches. All of this demonstrates several key points: (1) the importance of action in skill building—you cannot build skills without practicing those skills (i.e., taking action), and talking about skills is rarely sufficient; (2) that the concepts of collaborative motivation, framework consensus, and collaborative action are interrelated—in the example, Patricia's inability to move forward without the support and understanding of her therapist, her hopelessness, and her lack of motivation to do the work of therapy; and (3) that motivation, consensus, and action need to be addressed throughout therapy and flexibly deployed as the goals, tasks, and the client herself changes with treatment. Because the therapist continually checked in with Patricia, two common pitfalls were avoided, both of which can result in client demotivation: the client feeling overwhelmed by exercises that are beyond her skill/knowledge level or the client feeling bored by exercises that she has already mastered. In the case example of Patricia, the therapist made note of her progress in therapy, her increasing skill and ability to accept and manage her anxiety, and her motivation to continue pushing forward despite the increasing difficulty of the in-session practice pitches. Patricia felt validated and understood by the therapist in recognizing her accomplishments.

In the example of Patricia, the therapist conducted an assessment of Patricia's anxiety in order to understand the problem and how to move forward. The first exercises with the therapist as the audience could serve to assess Patricia's level of skill. Does she know that orienting the listener before launching into the pitch is advisable? Does she know to let the listener know a little about what they are going to hear before making the pitch and make sure to follow the pitch with a few concluding statements? Does Patricia know the basics of how speaking to an audience is different from speaking to friends or co-workers, one-on-one? Does Patricia know the value of talking slowly, taking deep breadths, repeating positive self-statements to herself, and other exercises to help her relax and focus before speaking in public? The assessment was therapeutic in that it generated a frame from which to proceed and addressed issues with motivation and collaborative action needed to get Patricia actively involved in solving the problem.

Whether the therapy is goal-oriented, insight-oriented, or simply supportive (or variations of these and other therapies), the process of talking, listening, and reflecting has the potential to help clients examine valuable material that may be related to their purpose for being in therapy and related to their hopes and dreams for the future. And regardless of type of therapy, achieving goals, gaining insight, and/or receiving and using support, consensus, and collaboration are essential to the process of healing. Consider the next case, masked and modified from a colleague's practice from several years ago.

Ivy, 41, came to therapy seeking help with her marriage, which was on the rocks. Her wife, Toni, had expressed dissatisfaction in their marriage and had recently confided in her that she was considering divorce. The issue, according to Toni, was that Ivy never talked about her feelings, what she wanted from their relationship, and, as a result, Toni felt less and less connected to Ivy over the years. Ivy agreed that this was a problem for her, but was always discouraged from discussing her feelings growing up and therefore she didn't feel comfortable doing so as an adult. When asked by the therapist what made it difficult for her to express her emotions, Ivy was at a loss. The therapist began by discussing with Ivy ideas for how therapy could benefit her, and they both explored the possibility that role-plays might help Ivy identify and express her feelings—first to the therapist and with time to Toni. Ivy agreed that this sounded like a good idea and that she understood how role-plays could serve as practice for her first forays into emotional expression. Ivy was able to identify that she still had strong, romantic feelings for Toni, a deep love and respect for her, but was also frustrated that Toni's expectations of her seem to have changed over the course of their relationship. The initial role-plays allowed the therapist and Ivy to recognize that Ivy's use of language might result in defensiveness, and they also identified Ivy's fears that expressing her emotions would cause Toni to reject her. Once Ivy and the therapist were able to discuss what was behind her difficulties in expressing her feelings to her spouse, they agreed to continue to practice together, in session, until she felt comfortable involving Toni. The therapist continually inquired with Ivy how she felt after each role-play and whether she felt ready to try something more difficult or found the role-play overwhelming. After a few weeks of practice with the therapist, Ivy invited Toni to the sessions and was able to express her fears and frustrations to her. While the therapist was more involved in the initial role-plays, her role became gradually less active. By the final few sessions, the therapist only provided the venue and an initial prompt, then sat back and allowed Ivy and Toni to speak.

The thoughtful reader can no doubt discern how this case could be approached conceptually and technically from a variety of theoretical and technical perspectives. The discussion that follows uses more of a problem-solving, cognitive-behavioral approach that involves individual and then couples therapy. In the preceding example, the therapist first had to understand why Ivy was unable to express herself emotionally to her spouse. Instead of asking Ivy about her difficulties, the therapist used role-play to have Ivy demonstrate her difficulties with emotional expression in real time. The therapist could also have used the emotional aspects of the here-and-now of the therapy relationship for the same purpose. What is important is that the therapist and client came to an understanding of Ivy's problems collaboratively. The causes of Ivy's difficulties with emotional expression were discovered together. With this information, the therapist was able to gradually guide Ivy to her desired destination, at the right tempo and level of intensity. If the therapist had moved Ivy too soon and too far ahead, Ivy could have felt that she was being asked to do something that was beyond her ability and that she was on her own (e.g., if the therapist had asked her to disclose some deep secret to Toni by herself after the first session). Conversely, if the therapist had moved along too slowly, Ivy would feel that the therapist doubted her ability to change and was in fact holding her back (e.g., not encouraging Ivy to practice her skills with Toni after she said she felt ready to do so).

Summary

Much has been written about and investigated using Bordin's conceptualization of the working alliance (i.e., agreement on the goals and tasks of therapy and the bond). It is indeed one of the most important ideas in the field of psychotherapy. We have discussed two broader, related concepts (i.e., *consensus* and *collaboration*) that we believe more correctly constitute the working alliance in therapy. And, consistent with the goal of this book, we have presented ways that counselors can go about establishing consensus and collaboration. In addition to discussing how consensus and collaboration evolve from the beginning to the end of therapy, we discussed three broad, significant, and pan-theoretical markers of consensus and collaboration: *collaborative motivation, framework consensus,* and *collaborative action.* We presented clinical examples of how these markers might manifest themselves in therapy and ways that they can be deliberately practiced in treatment. We hope that we have provided clinically oriented and useful material for in-session behavior for the reader, and we hope that we have stimulated further thinking about the nature of the working alliance in therapy.

References

Alexander, L. B., & Luborsky, L. (1987). The Penn Helping Alliance Scales. In L. S. Greenberg & W. M. Pinsoff (Eds.), *The psychotherapeutic process: A research handbook* (pp. 325–356). New York: Guilford.

Bedi, R. P., Davis, M. D., & Arvay, M. J. (2005). The client's perspective on forming a counselling alliance and implications for research on counsellor training. *Canadian Journal of Counselling, 39*(2), 71–85. Retrieved from http://ezproxy.library.ubc.ca/login?url=https://search-proquest-com.ezproxy.library.ubc.ca/docview/195803582?accountid=14656.

Bordin, E. S. (1979). The generalizability of the psychoanalytic concept of the working alliance. *Psychotherapy: Theory, Research, & Practice, 16,* 252–260.

Chow, D. L., Miller, S. D., Seidel, J. A., Kane, R. T., Thornton, J. A., & Andrews, W. P. (2015). The role of deliberate practice in the development of highly effective psychotherapists. *Psychotherapy, 52*(3), 337.345.

Egan, G. (2010). *The skilled helper: A problem management and opportunity development approach to helping* (9th ed.). Pacific Grove, CA: Brooks/Cole Cengage Learning.

Flückiger, C., Del Re, A. C., Wampold, B. E., & Horvath, A. O. (2018). The alliance in adult psychotherapy: A meta-analytic synthesis. *Psychotherapy.* Advance online publication. doi:10.1037/pst0000172

Gelso, C. J. (2006). Working alliance: Current status and future directions. *Psychotherapy: Theory, Research, Practice, Training, 43,* 257. doi:10.1037/0033-3204.43.3.257

Gelso, C. J., & Hayes, J. A. (1998). *The psychotherapy relationship: Theory, research, and practice.* New York: Wiley.

Gaston, L., & Marmar, C. (1994). The California Psychotherapy Alliance Scales. In A. O. Horvath & L. S. Greenberg (Eds.), *The working alliance: Theory, research, and practice* (pp. 85–108). New York: Wiley.

Goldberg, S. B., Babins-Wagner, R., Rousmaniere, T., Berzins, S., Hoyt, W. T., Whipple, J. L,. & Wampold, B. E. (2016). Creating a climate for therapist improvement: A case study of an agency focused on outcomes and deliberate practice. *Psychotherapy, 53*(3), 367–375.

Greene, J., Hibbard, J. H., Sacks, R., Overton, V., & Parrotta, C. D. (2015). When patient activation levels change, health outcomes and costs change, too. *Health Affairs (Millwood), 34,* 431–437.

Hatcher, R. L., & Barends, A. W. (1996). Patients' view of the alliance in psychotherapy: Exploratory factor analysis of three alliance measures. *Journal of Clinical and Consulting Psychology, 64,* 1326–1336.

Hatcher, R. L., & Barends, A. W. (2006). How a return to theory could help alliance research. *Psychotherapy: Theory, Research, Practice, Training, 43*, 292–299. doi:10.1037/0033-3204.43.3.292.

Hibbard, J. H., Mahoney, E. R., Stock, R., & Tusler, M. (2007). Do increases in patient activation result in improved self-management behaviors? *Health Services Research, 42*, 1443–1463.

Horvath, A. O., Del Re, AC, Flückiger, C., & Symonds, D. (2011). Alliance in individual psychotherapy. In J. C. Norcross (Ed.), *Psychotherapy relationships that work: Evidence-based responsiveness.* (2nd ed., pp. 25–69). New York; Oxford.

Horvath, A. O., & Greenberg, L. S. (1986). Development of the Working Alliance Inventory. In L. S. Greenberg & W. M. Pinsoff (Eds.), *The psychotherapeutic process: A research handbook* (pp. 529–556). New York: Guilford.

Lambert, M. J. (1992). Psychotherapy outcome research: Implications for integrative and eclectic therapists. In J. C. Norcross & M. R. Goldfried (Eds.), *Handbook of psychotherapy integration* (pp. 94–129). New York: Basic Books.

Miller, W. R., & Rollnick, S. (2012). *Motivational interviewing: Helping people change* (3rd ed.). New York: Guilford Press.

Norcross, J. C., & Lambert, M. J. (2018). Psychotherapy relationships that work III. *Psychotherapy, 55*, 303–315.

Norcross, J. C., & Wampold, B. E. (2011). Evidence-based therapy relationships: Research conclusions and clinical practices. *Psychotherapy, 48*, 98–102.

O'Malley, D., Dewan, A. A., Ohman-Strickland, P. A., Gundersen, D. A., Miller, S. M., & Hudson, S. V. (2018). Determinants of patient activation in a community sample of breast and prostate cancer survivors. *Psychooncology, 27*, 132–140.

O'Malley, S. S., Suh, C. S., & Strupp, H. H. (1983). The Vanderbilt Psychotherapy Process Scale: A report on the scale development and a process-outcome study. *Journal of Clinical and Consulting Psychology, 51*, 581–586.

Orlinsky, D. E., Rønnestad, M. H., &Willutzki, U. (2004). Fifty years of psychotherapy process- outcome research: Continuity and change. In M. J. Lambert (Ed.), *Bergin and Garfield's hand- book of psychotherapy and behavior change* (5th ed., pp. 307–390). Hoboken, NJ: Wiley.

Tryon, G. S., Birch, S. E.,& Verkuilen, J. (2018). Meta-analyses of the relation of goal consensus and collaboration to psychotherapy outcome. *Psychotherapy, 55*, 372–383.

6

Clients' Perspectives on, Experiences of, and Contributions to the Working Alliance

Implications for Clinicians

Robinder Bedi and Syler Hayes
University of British Columbia

Introduction and Overview

This chapter provides a practice-friendly overview of research related to clients' perspectives on, experiences of, and contributions to the working alliance, with implications for clinical practice. Specifically, this chapter aims to clarify the current state of knowledge about clients' understandings of the alliance and offer evidence-based suggestions for professionals to develop and maintain a working alliance that is responsive to clients' subjective understandings. Inevitably, there are no fully consistent findings on any aspect of alliance research. Therefore, presented here are the most likely conclusions and requisite implications of the current body of literature for mental health professionals based on the best available findings.

This chapter focuses on extrapolating from the results of the relatively few studies that allowed clients to present their own perspectives in an open-ended format. In contrast, the majority of alliance research has utilized psychometric measures, which are overwhelmingly premised on researchers' perspectives. Therefore, the conclusions within this chapter draw largely, but not entirely, on qualitative and mixed-methods research.

Clients frequently bring up variables beyond the parameters of the alliance models and theories most promoted by clinicians and researchers. Such variables include the experience of interventions as an extension of the relationship between the client and the clinician (e.g., Bedi, Davis, & Williams, 2005), the importance of validation and other counseling micro-skills (e.g., Bedi, 2006; MacFarlane, Anderson, & McClintock, 2015), and the impact of early interactions with clinicians and their office environment (e.g., Tryon, Blackwell, & Hammel, 2007). These factors are brought up even when the alliance has been specifically defined for clients in terms of Bordin's (1979) model and clients are prompted to specifically comment on contributors to developing a bond, a shared understanding of goals, and agreement on tasks (MacFarlane et al., 2015). The frequency with which these findings have been replicated led us to conclude that clients' experiences of the working alliance are dramatically different from clinicians' conventional understandings and experiences of the alliance (Bedi, 2006; Bedi & Richards, 2011).

Because clients' perspectives are underresearched, and many clinicians are unfamiliar with them, this chapter will provide extended attention to outlining clients' perspectives and experiences of the working alliance prior to providing concrete guidelines for practice. This chapter will use the terms "working alliance," "therapeutic alliance," and "alliance" interchangeably to match the mixed terminology of previous research studying this concept. This chapter is organized as follows. First, attention will be given to the importance of clients' perspective and experiences. Second, an overview will be provided on key research on clients' perspectives on, experiences of, and contributions to the working alliance. This section is divided into quantitative research and qualitative/mixed-methods research. Third, special attention is devoted to a client experience–focused theory of the alliance and client-identified alliance types. Fourth, the following relatively distinct features of clients' perspectives and experiences are presented and elaborated on: (a) alliance formation beginning prior to meeting the clinician and early in the first interaction (this includes the importance of the office environment in facilitating alliance formation), (b) the inseparability of clinical techniques and the therapeutic alliance, (c) the lack of collaboration that clients experience in alliance formation, (d) the importance of counseling micro-skills, and (e) the importance of validation in particular. Implications for clinician practice are embedded within each section. Finally, caveats and limitations for clinicians relying on the information synthesized in this chapter are presented.

Importance of Clients' Perspectives and Experiences

What the client brings to psychological treatment as a person and what the client does while in treatment matter and affect the success of counseling and psychotherapy more so than clinician-related variables such as the theories and techniques they employ (Asay & Lambert, 1999; Wampold, 2001; Wampold & Imel, 2015). In line with this, the latest meta-analysis of the association of the alliance with clinical outcome (Flückiger, Del Re, Wampold, & Horvath, 2018) replicates previous meta-analyses (e.g., Horvath & Bedi, 2002) and indicates that clients' ratings of the alliance are a better predictor of client outcome than are the ratings of mental health professionals. In other words, how the client experiences the alliance is the better indicator of the success of psychological treatment. Therefore, careful attention to clients' perspectives and experiences of the therapeutic alliance is warranted.

There is a tendency for clinicians to overestimate the extent to which they grasp clients' experiences. When clinicians are asked to recall the most significant moment for the client in a session, they only accurately identify what the client believes is most impactful about one-third of the time (Cummings, Martin, Hallbert, & Slemon, 1992; Martin & Stelmaczonek, 1988). Perspective discrepancies extend to the working alliance. In a meta-analytic examination of perspectives on the working alliance, client and clinician ratings of the working alliance were reported to have a correlation of only .36 (Tryon et al., 2007).

These apparent discrepancies cloud the existing body of research on the alliance. While there is ample research that claims to represent clients' perspectives and experiences of alliance formation and maintenance, most of it is based on the selection of variables theorized by researchers and clinicians. Previous researchers and clinicians have prioritized what they think is important for clients. However, these understandings are not always in line with what clients directly state themselves (i.e., with what they think is important). Using secondary means to try to comprehend clients' understandings and lived experiences limits our interpretations to those that fall within preexisting clinician and researcher assumptions (Bedi, 2006; Elliot & James, 1989). As a result, we know relatively little about how clients understand and experience the alliance or how the alliance forms relatively independently of the biasing lens of researchers and professionals (Bedi, Davis, & Arvay, 2005; Bedi, Davis, & Williams, 2005).

General Implications for Practice

Clinicians are encouraged to remember that clients' experiences of the alliance appear to be more important to successful counseling and psychotherapy than are their own (Flückiger et al., 2018). Therefore, clinicians are recommended to devote ample time to fostering the alliance throughout psychological treatment (i.e., not just at the outset), even when the clinician believes a strong alliance exists. In line with this, clinicians should guard against overconfidence in thinking they accurately understand what the client is experiencing (Smith & Agate, 2004) because clients commonly conceal their true feelings and often defer to what the clinician wants or expects (Rennie, 1994).

In addition, clinicians should be mindful of *confirmation bias* when they believe they understand how the client is experiencing the alliance and what the client thinks is the best way to develop and maintain it (Lilienfeld, Ritschel, Lynn, Cautin, & Latzman, 2014; Wright-McDougal & Toriello, 2013). To guard against confirmation bias, clinicians should seek out counterevidence to their clinical hypotheses for how to best develop/maintain an alliance with the client and remain open to testing out different interpersonal stances/strategies and evaluating the results (Lazarus, 1993). Moreover, clinicians are advised to regularly seek out feedback from the client about the strength of the working alliance, either verbally in session or formally through structured testing such as the Session Rating Scale (Duncan et al., 2003). Clients often appreciate the opportunity to disclose their difficulties with the treatment and the clinician when those experiences are acknowledged and validated (Miller, Duncan, Sorrell, & Brown, 2005), and therefore this strategy is also encouraged.

A Primer of Research on Clients' Perspectives on, Experiences of, and Contributions to the Alliance

The differences between clients' and clinicians' perspectives go well beyond mere differences in terminology whereby clinicians use psychological jargon and clients use lay terms. Instead, their entire conceptualizations of the alliance construct diverge in notable ways, such as perceiving different components of the alliance, valuing different variables for its formation, and subscribing to different theories for how it operates and creates positive outcomes.

Summary of Quantitative Research

Clients consistently rate the quality of the alliance higher than do their clinicians, especially those experiencing early success (Tryon et al., 2007). This can be problematic because research shows that when client and clinician ratings were inconsistent, even if one party rated psychotherapy highly, clinical outcomes were hindered (Zilcha-Mano et al., 2016). This difference may be partially due to clinicians having more experience with the working alliance and thus being able to draw on a larger set of experiences (Zilcha-Mano et al., 2016). This difference may also partially be due to clients relying on early outcomes as a sign of the alliance, whereas clinicians more commonly consider the alliance and outcome to be conceptually distinct (Zilcha-Mano et al., 2016).

Indeed, quantitative research frequently indicates that clients' views on the working alliance are more closely tied to the perceived benefit of the treatment (i.e., feeling helped)—that is, the separation of alliance and outcome is much less distinct in the minds of clients than clinicians (Hatcher, Barends, Hansell, & Gutfreund, 1995). In other words, psychological treatment may need to be experienced as somewhat helpful for the client before the client will rate the working alliance as strong. In addition, clinicians are also prone to overestimate the strength of clients' ratings about the helpfulness of the clinician and the treatment (e.g., Hartmann, Joos, Orlinsky, & Zeeck, 2015). Given the close association clients make between the perceived benefit of treatment and what clinicians refer to as the alliance, this would logically translate into a misunderstanding of the strength of the alliance from the clients' perspectives.

In this manner, many clients' experiences and perspectives closely fit Luborsky's (1976) model of the alliance. In Luborsky's two-type sequential model, *type I alliance* refers to a warm, supportive relationship that the client experiences as *helpful*, and a *type II alliance* refers to client investment in the process and shared responsibility for outcome. Somewhat further distancing themselves from Bordin's (1979) conceptualization, clients often make less conscious differentiations between the goals of psychological treatment and the tasks that are designed to meet these goals (Hatcher & Barends, 1996, 2006). Frequently observed high correlations between the goals and task subscales of the client version of the Working Alliance Inventory also challenge the separation of these two (out of three) pillars of Bordin's model (Hatcher & Barends, 1996, 2006) for describing how clients experience the working alliance.

Moreover, factor analyses of measures of the alliance, purportedly tapping into clients' experiences, identify underlying dimensions that are discrepant with popular alliance theories, such as confident collaboration, idealized relationship, and help received (Hatcher & Barends, 1996, 2006). This discrepancy has led some to conclude that, when it comes to the alliance, clients experience much more than and in a different manner than clinicians (Hatcher & Barends, 1996, 2006). In connecting this to Bordin's theory, Hatcher and Barends (1996) state that clients develop a bond based on effective therapeutic work and confidence in the collaboration. However, they point to the need for substantial revising of existing alliance measures to better capture clients' perspectives.

Implications for Practice

Clinicians should recognize that they are likely misunderstanding the strength of the alliance that the client is experiencing, and this could partly be because they are overestimating the degree of helpfulness that the client is experiencing. Therefore, clinicians should continually and directly seek explicit client feedback to compare against their own observations, even when treatment appears to be going smoothly (Kivlighan, Marmaroth, & Hilsenroth, 2014). The research can be taken to suggest that clinicians need to spend more time trying to accurately evaluate the strength of the alliance, in collaboration with the client, and try to come to an honest, mutually agreeable understanding, especially in early interactions when initial expectations are being developed and tested (Zilcha-Mano et al., 2016). For example, a clinician could say something like, "everyone is different and what works for one individual can be quite different from what works for another; because we've only just started to get to know each other, I'm just wondering what's going well in our working relationship and what I could be doing differently?" Alternately, a clinician could utilize brief process-oriented measures, such as the Session Rating Scale (Duncan et al., 2003), and discuss them with the client at the next session.

Resolving disagreements about and clarifying expectations for the eventual process of psychological treatment is further recommended because successfully doing so may further strengthen the alliance (Zilcha-Mano et al., 2016). In many cases, clients should be directly asked about what they expect from psychological treatment at the present time, and a frank discussion should be had about what the professional can and cannot reasonably offer. Clients cannot always answer these questions or may be unwilling to do so early in the process. As such, it also seems important to explore the answers to questions indirectly by speaking to clients' current expectations: "Have you ever seen a counselor and psychologist before, and what was that experience like?" "What did you like and not like as much about your last counselor?" "What do you know about what happens in a counseling session?" "What do you think about how therapy is portrayed on television and movies?" And, "do you know anyone else who has gone to counseling and what was that like for them?" In some situations, clients' expectations may be unrealistic, be based on misunderstandings of what psychological treatment is and how it works, or be beyond the training and capabilities of the particular clinician. But having open and direct conversations about these discrepancies, if handled with honesty, respect, and humility, can sometimes help to create a great sense of collaboration (Crits-Christoph, Gibbons, & Hearon, 2006).

In addition, clinicians should be mindful that, although they are typically taught that clinical outcome is a wholly distinct concept from the working alliance, this is not typically the case in the minds of clients. Clients appear to base their perceptions of the quality of the overall working alliance on the perceived helpfulness of the therapeutic work. Although this is somewhat of an oversimplification, we can expect clients who are experiencing early benefits from psychological treatment to feel closer to and bond better with the clinician, to be more willing to agree with clinician-suggested therapeutic tasks, and to collaborate or compromise more willingly on therapeutic goals. If the client believes that the clinician will be or has been helpful, positive relational consequences will result, including for the alliance (Puschner, Wolf, & Kraft, 2008). In support of this notion of the effectiveness of counseling and psychotherapy being tied to the quality of the alliance (Luborsky, 1976; Zilcha-Mano et al. 2016), there is a small body of literature that demonstrates that early clinical outcomes subsequently contribute to higher ratings of the working alliance (Crits-Christoph et al., 2006; Crits-Christoph, Gibbons, Hamilton, Ring-Kurtz, & Gallop, 2011) rather than just the other way around. In addition to directly asking the client about how effective treatment is and collaboratively assessing progress toward client-stated goals, standardized measures of outcome can be useful (e.g., the Outcome Questionnaire-45; Lambert, Gregersen, & Burlingame, 2004), including when they are discussed in session with the client and the client is given the opportunity to agree, disagree, and ask questions.

A similar conflation occurs in the minds of clients for goals and tasks. Clients may not experience or appreciate the distinction in session as much as clinicians do. Clinicians should be cognizant that, despite whatever concept of the alliance they are using to structure their understanding (e.g., Bordin's goals, tasks, bond), the client is likely not using this same framework and may in fact be drawing on a different understanding of the alliance. Therefore, clinicians should generally refrain from inflexibly promoting their own particular view of the working alliance onto the client. Instead, clinicians should treat their conceptualization of the alliance as a hypothesis with each client, seeking both confirmatory and disconfirmatory evidence as well as being aware about alternative conceptualizations of the alliance and considering them in the same manner. Evidence can be gleaned directly from what clients say about the working alliance (noting that they may refer to it as a "working relationship"; Bedi, Davis, & Williams, 2005), either when asked directly or when talking spontaneously about it.

Summary of Qualitative and Mixed-Methods Research

A Client Theory of Alliance

Only one major theory of the alliance has been proposed that has been solidly grounded in clients' unimpeded reported lived experiences. A Positive Emotion-Exploration/Negative Emotion-Lack of Exploration Spiral Theory has been proposed to explain the nature of the alliance from clients' perspectives and its connection to therapeutic outcome (Bedi, Cook, & Domene, 2012; Fitzpatrick, Janzen, Chamodraka, & Park, 2006; Fitzpatrick, Janzen, Chamodraka, Gamberg, & Blake, 2009).

According to this theory, in order to develop and grow the alliance, the process begins with the client ascribing favorable meaning to a particular clinician behavior or verbalization and experiencing positive affect. A positive client understanding and experience can be the result of, for example, the clinician asking an intriguing question, offering a new way to look at an issue, providing useful psycho-education or psychological skills training, permitting the client unfettered verbal or emotional expression, making an appreciated self-disclosure, complimenting the client, or reassuring the client (Fitzpatrick et al., 2006). For example, the clinician could say something like, "Have you ever looked at it this way . . . ?," or "there's a lot of people who've gone through this and made it through," "I can tell how hard of a worker you are," or "it was really hard for me when I went through something similar." In return, the client may think something constructive and affirmative such as "my therapist can help me" or "I'm important" (Fitzpatrick et al., 2006, p. 491) and experience positive affect. As a result of this positive affect, the client then responds with increased openness to deeper exploration through both self-disclosure (i.e., productive openness) and making use of input from the clinician (i.e., receptive openness). For example, the client may then say: "for the first time this session, I was talking about something really hard to hear and even to talk about" or "I was very open. I wasn't knocking things down" (Fitzpatrick et al., 2006, p. 491). Being open can result in further positive feelings and inspire further openness, which then can lead to further positive feelings and so on. In other words, it is theorized that client openness to exploration, combined with positive emotional responses to the clinician's actions, results in the initial development of the working alliance and its subsequent strengthening. It can be further postulated that through this client openness, progress is made in counseling and psychotherapy, and therefore the alliance should be associated with clinical outcome.

According to this theory, alliance development and strengthening is premised on client openness and positive emotions. Connecting this theory with Bordin's (1979) model, positive feelings on the part of the client contribute to bonding with the clinician, which then subsequently leads to greater openness and exploration, which results in shared goals and agreement on tasks to achieve those goals (Fitzpatrick et al., 2009).

In contrast, a negative downward spiral can also account for diminished alliances and alliance ruptures (Bedi et al., 2012; Fitzpatrick et al., 2006). In this case, the client interprets and then reacts to something that the clinician said or did with negative feelings that impede additional exploration and openness. For example, in response to a clinician being highly directive, stating something factually incorrect, or looking distracted, the client may react by not telling the professional what the client was really thinking or minimize the severity of the problem (Bedi et al., 2012). This, in turn, predictably prompts additional negative affect in the client, which leads to further reduced exploration and openness, which creates more negative affect, following a decreasing spiral and reducing the quality of the working alliance.

In Richards and Bedi (2015), decrements in the alliance with male clients were the most associated with rigidly adhering to a therapeutic approach that was "not the right fit" (p. 170). In other words, these approaches were incongruent with the client's understanding of what was helpful, important, appropriate, or related. As evidence, clients in their study said things such as (a) "the counselor and I did 'weird' exercises to address my issues that I thought were a waste of time" and (b) "the counselor suggested that her way—her philosophies and method of healing—were the only way that would work" (Richards & Bedi, 2015; p. 176). Based on research by Coutinho, Ribeiro, Hill, and Safran (2011), it was concluded that there are a wide variety of precipitants of alliance ruptures from clients' perspectives. The examples they found in their study included the professional doing or saying things that the client did not like, such as providing unsolicited advice, talking about a painful topic with the client before the client was ready; or failing to do something the client wanted, such as not remembering something the client previously said. About 19–37% of clients experience significant ruptures in the alliance with their professional (Eames & Roth, 2000; Muran, Safran, Samstag, & Winston, 2005), about 30% of which remained unresolved in the client's opinion (Coutinho et al., 2011). Often, clients do not directly inform their clinicians about this weakening of the alliance (Rhodes, Hill, Thompson, & Elliot, 1994). Although, as noted earlier, the specific content of alliance ruptures can be quite variable across clients, it appears that the impact on clients' experiences is fairly consistent. As a result of an experienced rupture, clients typically feel sad, helpless, abandoned, criticized, or confused. For example, in response to an alliance-rupturing event, clients have said (a) "I felt very angry when the therapist suggested I do different activities because the therapist knew all the problems I had at home. So, it was like telling a paraplegic to walk"; and (b) "when the therapist suggested to do something different, I got confused. It was very hard to see things in a way I never saw before. It seemed I was losing my identity" (Coutinho et al., 2011, p. 534).

Implications for Practice

Clinicians should stay alert to and respond to ongoing clients' negative affect in session (explicit or implied), noting that it is likely indicative of a weakened alliance or full-blown alliance rupture. Sometimes paying careful attention to momentary client facial responses can cue the clinician that a hindering event has occurred (Barros, Altimir, & Perez, 2016). Given that clients often keep this information secret (Coutinho et al., 2011), it is recommended that clinicians persist in their exploration of negative affect in session and engage the client in an explicit and active discussion about the working alliance and ways to improve it. This can be accomplished in various ways. For example, a clinician could use immediacy and share the clinician's awareness of the client's potentially problematic nonverbal behavior, such as avoiding eye contact, crossed arms, turning away from the clinician, and rolling eyes. A clinician could also directly ask the client to discuss negative emotions in the moment if the clinician believes that a rupture has occurred or if the client expresses negativity (Safran & Muran, 2000). The clinician can then respond in an empathetic manner rather than with defensiveness (Safran & Muran, 2000). Something that a clinician could specifically say is, "I noticed that your responses to me are much less detailed after I asked if you had told your partner about your changing values, and I'm curious what shifted after my questions."

Research shows that clinicians rarely do anything different when the client experiences a rupture and instead often continue as if nothing had happened (Coutinho et al., 2011). In some cases, they are unaware of the rupture, but many times they are aware but continue in the same manner because they do not know what to do (Coutinho et al., 2011). Instead, clients typically want the clinician to change strategies and do something different, particularly as many ruptures are repetitions of previous ruptures (Coutinho et al., 2011). Clients in the Coutinho et al. (2011) study also reported wishing for more guidance from the clinician about what to do to resolve the rupture, wanting the clinician to express interest in the client as a person, and wanting more empathy for their heightened emotional states, even when they were confrontational toward the clinician. Therefore, it is also recommended that clinicians bring up and openly discuss ruptures in the alliance and explicitly offer suggestions on resolving them, all the while remembering to express care and concern about the person and empathize with any negative feelings and/or reactions toward the clinician (Coutinho et al., 2011; Safran, Muran, & Eubanks-Carter, 2011). A clinician might say something such as, "Now that you've mentioned it, I can totally understand your frustration at me not noticing the small but very important changes you've made this week. I should have noticed and mentioned them but I was too focused on trying to push you to go further. Can we take a few minutes to discuss what is the best balance of challenge and support/acknowledgment that will help you get the most of our work together? Helping me figure this out will help us work together more effectively and prevent me from making the same mistake over and over again."

Client Alliance Types

From clients' perspectives, the alliance can be conceptualized according to two different typologies. It can either be conceived of across the personal–professional dimension (Mohr & Woodhouse, 2000, 2001) or as one of three distinct kinds: nurturant, insight-oriented, or collaborative (Bachelor, 1995).

A personal alliance is one characterized by warmth, a deep emotional connection, a nonthreatening working relationship, and mutual self-disclosure (Mohr & Woodhouse, 2000, 2001). For example, clients have said "something that turned me on to my current therapist is how down-to-earth, caring, respectful and honest he is with me. He has no problem telling me why my day was bad or why he is pissed off. . . . I honestly can say that when you can call your therapist one of your best friends, it is critical" (Mohr & Woodhouse, 2001, p. 16). In contrast, a professional alliance is characterized by stronger personal boundaries, impartiality, explicit collaboration, and a working relationship where the clinician challenges the client and facilitates deeper exploration and insight. For example, clients have said, "I am not quite comfortable with the 'I am your friend, I feel your pain' approach. . . . I pay you. . . . While I understand the need of genuine concern in therapy, it is not always helpful. I'd like a therapist to be two steps ahead of me" (p. 16). Most clients' expectations likely fall somewhere in between these two extremes. Extant research suggests that most clients prefer elements in line with a personal alliance (Bedi & Duff, 2009).

Alternatively, alliances can be understood as either primarily nurturant, insight-oriented, or collaborative (Bachelor, 1995). A nurturant alliance centers on warmth, friendliness, active listening, patience, and strong empathic understanding—similar to the classic person-centered approach (Rogers, 1961). In a nurturant alliance, the client might say "she's truly a friend for me. . . . I feel her to be attentive, sensitive, available, listening. . . . I trust her entirely" (Bachelor, 1995, p. 336). An insight-oriented alliance centers on the exploratory nature of the therapeutic work, with the clinician focused on explicit guidance, keeping the client on track, and both facilitating greater client self-expression and helping the client achieve greater self-understanding than clients can on their own. In an insight-oriented alliance, the client could say, "she makes me talk a lot and I feel intensely all the emotions that she makes me experience. . . . I am surprised by what she is able to make me say, because often these are things which I had forgotten or not suspected as being a problem" (p. 336). A collaborative alliance centers on equality, two-way active involvement, and mutuality. In a collaborative alliance, the client can say "she told me that it wouldn't be her who would find my problems but us together" and "the exchange . . . consists of mutual verbal exploration of the situation, of exchanging, and mutual evaluation of solutions" (p. 336). It is unclear what most clients expect. Bachelor's (1995) study found the highest prevalence rate for a nurturant alliance (46%), while the two studies contained within Bedi and Duff (2009) found insight-oriented (52%) and collaborative (54%) to be most prevalent, respectively, with nurturant the least common in both samples. When asked directly, it appears that clients prefer the triadic typology of Bachelor's over Mohr and Woodhouse's dyadic typology in conceptualizing the alliance (Bedi & Duff, 2009).

Implications for Practice
Based on the preceding information, it is recommended that clinicians develop a highly malleable and flexible interpersonal stance. In a sense, they may need to become, relationally, "an authentic chameleon" (Lazarus, 1993, p. 404) in order to tailor their relational stance to provide the working relationship of choice for the particular client at hand (Norcross & Beutler, 1997). For example, some clients may wish to hear about the clinician's personal life and maintain more

of an alliance that represents some aspects of a close friendship, while others consider this harmful to the alliance (Mohr & Woodhouse, 2000). Clinicians should, early in treatment, attempt an assessment of the client's preferred relational stance based on the preceding dimensions or categories. Because no formal, well-accepted psychometric measure exists (to our knowledge) that assesses client relational preferences, this will likely have to be done through less standardized means. One manner is to ask about the client's relationship with a previous clinician ("So how did you get along with your previous counsellor and what worked and didn't work?). Another is to identify significant relational patterns in the client's life and relate them to psychological treatment (e.g., "I have noticed that you really respect your friends who tell it to you like it is; that is, they don't hold back telling you the truth, and I am guessing that this approach will be helpful for me to take on."). Of course, this can also be done through a combination of (a) asking clients directly (e.g., "Is it better that I spend more time listening and trying hard to understand what you're going through or would you rather I just jump in with any insights that I think I might have?") and (b) appraising early interactions with clients for their reactions (e.g., does the client respond more or go deeper after a clinician self-disclosure versus when confronted about an inconsistency between their words and actions?). The clinician should keep in mind that these are tendencies, and clients may resemble more than one type and change their preference over time (Bachelor, 1995). Clinicians should therefore remain watchful and continually reassess the expectations of the client.

Distinct Features of Clients' Perspectives and Experiences

As noted earlier, professionals' understandings of the alliance can diverge substantially from clients' understandings. Some key ways that clients' perspectives and lived experiences are at odds with those of professionals and deviate from the conclusions of most alliance researchers revolve around pretreatment and initial interactions, the office environment, the techniques–alliance interface, collaboration, clinician micro-skills, and the prominence of validation over other micro-skills.

Initial and Early Interactions and the Environmental Context

Before attending treatment, many clients have initial reservations (MacFarlane et al., 2015). These preconceptions are developed in a variety of ways, including through popular media representations (MacFarlane et al., 2015), and can support or impair the initial development of the alliance. Even before meeting their clinicians, clients have been found to extrapolate their impressions from their initial interactions with front office staff, which can make it easier or more difficult for the clinician to subsequently develop an alliance with the client (Bedi, 2006; Bedi, Davis, & Williams, 2005). In addition, clients also seem to create quick impressions based on their initial and early interactions with the clinician by things as seemingly innocuous as clinician attire, clinician grooming, the manner by which the clinician greets the client (e.g., warmly, by name), appropriately firm handshakes, and whether or not the clinician recognizes the client in the waiting room (Bedi, 2006; Bedi, Davis, & Arvay, 2005; Bedi, Davis, & Williams, 2005). For example, clients have said, (a) "my counselor always seemed happy to see me, greeting me with warmth" (Simpson & Bedi, 2012, p. 361) and (b) "the psychotherapist recognized me (remembered my name, made eye contact with me while I was in the waiting room)" (Bedi & Richards, 2011, p. 384).

Furthermore, at the outset of the first session, clients typically scan the office environment and make judgments about the clinician based on factors such as the tidiness of the clinician's desk, the nature of books on shelves, the lighting and colors of the office, and the comfort of chairs (Bedi, 2006; Bedi, Davis, & Arvay, 2005; Bedi, Davis, & Williams, 2005). For example, clients have said, (a) "you want to see it as a professional place and not dirty and grungy. You want to see that the person cares about the office. The office helps make you feel comfortable" and (b) "I was surprised at the importance I'd put on setting. . . . For my own experience, in looking back, I see how it had a profound influence on my feeling safe to continue with my counselor" (Bedi, 2006, p. 32). These initial experiences then reportedly also predispose clients toward developing working alliances with professionals in an easier or more difficult manner (Bedi, 2006; Bedi, Davis, & Arvay, 2005; Bedi, Davis, & Williams, 2005; Simpson & Bedi, 2012). So, in the minds of clients, alliance formation actually begins before the professional first meets the client. Fortunately, there is slowly growing recognition from clinicians about the importance of the office environment and other contextual factors in impacting clients (e.g., Benton & Overtree, 2012; Borenstein, 2006; Devlin et al., 2009; Devlin & Nasar, 2012; Miya & Hanyu, 2006; Nasar & Devlin, 2011).

Implications for Practice
Clinicians should inform their office staff how vital of a role they play in client success. The better the impression and experience the client has with the front staff and the physical reception area, the easier it will be for the client and clinician to quickly develop a solid working alliance. Therefore, clinicians should appropriately thank the support staff and, if possible, work with support staff and

administrators to ensure that the initial impression of the physical space is likely to be inclusive and welcoming.

In addition, the clinician should be mindful of the apparent importance of first impressions created at the outset of psychological treatment and at the start of every session. Research implicates the importance of devoting time early in treatment to understanding and working through initial misgivings that clients may have about psychological treatment. It is therefore recommended that clinicians, each session but especially the first one, show recognition of the client if there was previous contact, warmly greet the client by name, and groom and dress well. Furthermore, clinicians should take extra effort to structure their office to create the type of impression that they wish to portray as well as maximize the comfort of clients. Clients do not usually offer this type of information willingly, even when prompted (Blanchard & Farber, 2016). Clinicians will likely need to initiate the discussion, take initial client responses with "a grain of salt" (because clients may not initially be forthright), engage in assessment based on something other than clients' direct responses, and revisit the topic as needed. One thing a clinician could say would be, "I sometimes worry about the first impression that I can create on the days that I am so busy that I don't have time to tidy up my desk." Another thing is, "It's pretty common for individuals to develop quick impressions of their counselors. Now that we've been working together for a while, I am curious to know your thoughts and feelings about our work together so far?"

Techniques Versus Working Alliance

Clients' understandings of the alliance seem to challenge the frequently used distinction among therapists between techniques and therapeutic alliance (Mohr & Woodhouse, 2001). Psychotherapy strategies and interventions are central to clients' accounts of alliance formation (Bedi, 2006; Bedi, Davis, & Arvay, 2005; Bedi, Davis, & Williams, 2005; Bedi & Richards, 2011; Fitzpatrick et al., 2006, 2009; Simpson & Bedi, 2012) and reduced alliance quality (Bedi et al., 2012; Richards & Bedi, 2015). For example, Bedi, Davis, and Williams (2005) found that clients frequently note specific clinical techniques as responsible for alliance formation. In this study, most examples of client-identified alliance formation related to clinician technical activity. Additionally, most clients also reported technical activity as key to their alliance formation. Similarly, Bedi, Davis, and Arvay (2005) found that general counseling skills was both the largest category of client-identified alliance formation variables as well as the most prevalent one across clients in their sample, being noted by every single one of the clients in their study. In research by Bedi (2006), clinician technical activity revolving around teaching the client skills, assigning clinical homework, and psycho-education was the second highest rated category of client-identified alliance formation factors, only behind the category of "validation."

In Fitzpatrick et al.'s (2006, 2009) research, clinician technical interventions that promoted alliance development were ones that helped clients think or act in a new way, encouraged clients to take space, demonstrated interest, provided emotional support, communicated understanding, demonstrated nonjudgmental attitudes, shared something meaningful (such as compliments, reassurance, positive feedback, tools, or assignments), or met clients' unexpressed needs. Bedi and Richards (2011) found that when a male client experienced practical help from the clinician, this correlated largely with Working Alliance Inventory – Short Form revised total scores ($r = .41$). Other evidence consistent with the claim that techniques can facilitate the alliance include (a) Luborsky's (1976) findings that psychodynamic interpretations, if suitable, resulted in improved alliances while unsuitable ones had the opposite effect and (b) Kivlighan's (1990) finding that technical activity accounted for 32% of the variation in clients' ratings of the working alliance.

Whereas a clinician implements a particular clinical technique with the intention of impacting outcomes positively (i.e., helping the client get better), in the minds of clients, these interventions have significant relational implications that can override the outcome-focused intention of the professional (Bedi, Davis, & Arvay, 2005; Bedi, Davis & Williams, 2005). The clinician may not be offering a particular intervention with the goal of fostering the working alliance with the client, but that is what often occurs from the client's perspective. Therefore, to clients, clinical techniques serve the additional function of alliance-formation strategies when delivered in a manner that makes the client feel cared for, respected, and hopeful (Fitzpatrick et al., 2006, 2009).

Implications for Practice

Clinical interventions are often understood by clients as having relational consequences for the formation, strengthening, and maintenance of the alliance beyond their direct impact on outcome. So, in the minds of clients, techniques cannot be divorced from the context of the working alliance and neither should they be for clinicians. When deciding on an intervention, clinicians should be aware that the client is likely looking at the suggestion and implementation of the intervention through a relational lens. The process and outcome of the intervention will likely provide feedback to the client about the nature and quality of the working alliance between the client and clinician.

Collaboration

Collaboration is well-regarded in predominant alliance theories as one of the foundational components of the alliance (Bordin, 1979; Hatcher & Barends, 1996). In contrast, the most replicated finding across research on clients' perspectives on and experiences of the alliance is that clients do not characteristically reaffirm the collaborative nature of alliance formation and maintenance. Instead, clients highlight clinical contributions as the engine of alliance formation and place the primary responsibility for alliance formation on clinicians (Bachelor, 1995; Bedi, 2006; Bedi & Duff, 2014; Bedi & Richards, 2011; Bedi, Davis, & Arvay 2005; Bedi, Davis, & Williams, 2005; Bedi et al., 2012; Duff & Bedi, 2010; Fitzpatrick et al., 2006, 2009; MacFarlane et al., 2015; Mohr & Woodhouse, 2001; Simpson & Bedi, 2012). Clinicians should not necessarily expect clients to be initially thinking about therapeutic collaboration as clients often enter treatment in great psychological distress, feeling incompetent in resolving their problems, and "unable to handle much responsibility" (Bedi, 2006, p. 32).

Implications for Practice

Despite collaboration not being a core phenomenological experience of clients, clients do not have to identify or experience what they are doing in alliance formation and maintenance as collaborative for it to actually be collaboration in some objective manner (Hatcher & Barends, 2006). In other words, clients often do not readily identify what they are doing as collaboration or notice their own contributions to the alliance. A small amount of research indicates that, as sessions progress, later in psychological treatment, clients tend to take on more agency in maintaining the alliance (e.g., Fitzpatrick et al., 2009) and that men might be more collaborative early in treatment (Bedi & Richards, 2011). Nevertheless, clients can sometimes recognize greater collaborative self-involvement in the alliance with direct probing (Fitzpatrick et al., 2009). In counseling and psychotherapy, understanding how client participation can help or hinder the development and maintenance of the alliance could be quite therapeutic for clients in and of itself, as well as improve the working alliance directly (Fitzpatrick et al., 2006).

Therefore, it is recommended that clinicians focus clients' attention on the collaborative nature of the alliance and perhaps educate them on the need for mutual responsibility and effort in creating a successful working relationship— in a sense, demystifying the process (MacFarlane et al., 2015). For example, a clinician can say something such as, "A relationship takes two people to work— and this includes the working relationship between me and you. We really need to work together to be most effective. I will always try what has been successful for most people I have worked with but everyone is different—and what has worked for someone else may not necessarily work for you. So we really need to put both of our heads together and combine our wisdom and experience." This idea is completely in line with the larger principle underlying role induction techniques, which have been shown to improve client engagement and prevent clients' unilateral termination (Swift & Greenberg, 2015). Role induction can be accomplished simply by giving the client a handout on what counseling or psychotherapy is and what to expect or by spending 5 minutes telling the client what the clinician expects and what the client should expect of the clinician (and then processing it and coming to a mutual understanding).

Counseling Micro-Skills

Forming the alliance may be deceptively simple and centered on counseling micro-skills (Bedi, 2006; Bedi, Davis, & Arvay, 2005; Bedi, Davis & Williams, 2005; MacFarlane et al., 2015). However, these micro-skills may be so ubiquitous that professionals may fail to fully appreciate their potentially powerful impact on the alliance. Clients frequently note the pivotal importance of nonverbal and paraverbal skills, such as the SOLER physical attending skills (face the client Squarely, Open posture, Leaning in slightly, Eye contact, and Relaxed posture), head nodding, paraverbal prompts (e.g. "uh-huh," "mm-hmmm," "yes," "okay"), smiling, and shared laughter (e.g., Bedi, Davis, & Arvay, 2005). Clients also frequently acknowledge as integral the pivotal importance of nonjudgmental, active listening verbal skills, especially for initial alliance formation: identifying and reflecting feelings/empathic reflections, paraphrases/content reflections, summaries, validation, normalization, and complimenting the client/pointing out client strengths (Bachelor, 1995; Bedi, 2006; Bedi et al., 2012; Bedi, Davis. & Arvay, 2005; Bedi, Davis, & Williams, 2005; Bedi & Duff, 2009, 2014; Bedi & Richards, 2011; Duff & Bedi, 2010; Fitzpatrick et al., 2006, 2009; MacFarlane et al., 2015; Mohr & Woodhouse, 2001; Richards & Bedi, 2015; Simpson & Bedi, 2012). Such research findings even hold up when the alliance was overtly defined for clients in line with Bordin's (1979) definition. Clients still listed these micro-skills as essential for the bond, goals, and tasks components of the alliance (MacFarlane et al., 2015).

To further highlight the importance of counseling micro-skills, presented here is a collection of sample quotations from clients concerning what they identified as important for alliance formation and maintenance as related to the above-mentioned micro-skills:

1. "The therapist made eye contact while listening to me" (Bedi, Davis, & Williams, 2005, p. 318).
2. "The way my counsellor sat, moved etc. indicated that he was comfortable and he was not somehow personally threatened, closed-off, or upset" (Simpson & Bedi, 2012, p. 357).
3. "The therapist remembered and repeated back things that I had said in previous sessions" (Bedi, Davis, & Williams, 2005, p. 318).
4. "The therapist recognized my feelings and put a name to them when I couldn't" (Bedi, Davis, & Williams, 2005, p. 318).
5. "The therapist normalized my feelings saying 'this happens to couples' and 'that happened to me, too'" (Bedi, Davis, & Williams, 2005, p. 319).
6. "The psychotherapist identified and reflected back my feelings" (Bedi & Richards, 2011, p. 384).
7. "The counselor did not judge me and made me feel like everything I was dealing with was normal" (Simpson & Bedi, 2012, p. 357).
8. "My counselor took my perceptions and beliefs at face value without putting his meaning on my experience. My counsellor worked with me, not the counselor's story of me" (Simpson & Bedi, 2012, p. 361).
9. "My counselor always seemed happy to see me, greeting me with warmth and a solid hug. She commented on my strengths as an individual and expressed heartfelt happiness when things in my life were going well" (Simpson & Bedi, 2012, p. 361).
10. "I felt it was very easy talking to my therapist because he gave a sense that he was understanding my feelings" (MacFarlane et al., 2015, p. 367).
11. "I brought forward this issue . . . and we covered that first and then she let me sort of explain, she was very unobtrusive and she let me get it all off my chest" (Fitzpatrick et al., 2006, p. 491).
12. "We talked about something and she related it to something in my life that I had already told her and it was . . . a connection that I had never made" (Fitzpatrick et al., 2009, p. 568).

Although it is not without its limitations, the micro-skills approach has become the dominant paradigm for counselor training (McLennan, 1994; Ridley, Kelly, & Mollen, 2011). There is an abundance of research that shows the effectiveness of counseling micro-skills (e.g., Kim & Kim, 2013), including in randomized control trials of facilitative interpersonal skills (e.g., Anderson et al., 2016). Notably, even entire training textbooks have been grounded in the micro-skills approach (e.g., Daniels & Ivey, 2007). Fortunately, such skills are highly trainable (Levitt, 2002; Kuntze, van der Molen, & Born, 2009).

In Bedi and Richards (2011), clinician nonverbal behaviors correlated .33 to .46 with the total Working Alliance Inventory – Short Form, revised (WAI-Sr) and its subscales of goals, tasks, and bond, with the highest correlation with the tasks subscale. Duff and Bedi (2010) found moderate to high correlations between clinician eye contact, greeting the client with a smile, referring to details discussed in previous sessions, clinician responding honestly, clinician sitting still without fidgeting, and clinician facing the client and alliance as measured by the WAI-Sr. Duff and Bedi's (2010) study further demonstrated that what clients believe to influence alliance development is supported by quantitative research.

Implications for Practice

Although one can easily be seduced by advanced theoretical conceptualizations of the client and of the alliance, as well as by the plethora of clinical techniques available, clients' reports frequently make note of basic counseling micro-skills as essential for developing and maintaining the working alliance. Therefore, it is recommended that clinicians make frequent use of the micro-skills noted here—not only at the outset of psychological treatment to develop the alliance but throughout it to maintain the alliance, especially after ruptures occur.

Validation

Of all the counseling micro-skills, validation appears to play the most prominent role as reported by clients. Researchers studying clients' perspectives have defined validation as communicating to the client that their experiences are not abnormal and that they are legitimate or defensible (Bedi, Davis, & Williams, 2005). Duff and Bedi (2010) stated that validation was grounded in the clinician's positive regard and liking of the client (Rogers, 1961). In their own words, by validation, clients mean that a clinician "[said] that my reaction was understandable and reasonable, that it was okay to feel this way," "normalized my experience," "made encouraging comments," "made positive comments about me," and "agreed with what I said" (Bedi, 2006, p. 31). Validation can also be accomplished by appropriate clinician self-disclosure, as noted by the client who stated that validation occurred when the counselor said, "That happened to me, too" (Bedi, Davis, & Williams, 2005, p. 319).

Although validation of clients' experiences is already highly regarded in the psychological treatment literature (Linehan, 1997), in the minds of clients, it seems to be one of the most important variables for alliance formation. Some research shows that it can actually be more potent than empathic verbal reflections, particularly in increasing client self-esteem and elevating low client mood (Kim & Kim, 2013). In Bedi, Davis, and Williams (2005), validation was one of the more prevalent categories of client-identified alliance formation factors. In Bedi (2006), validation was the highest rated category of client-identified alliance formation factors. In Duff and Bedi (2010), validation, defined as making encouraging comments, making positive comments about the client, and greeting the client with a smile, accounted for 62% of the variance in client-rated working alliance scores (WAI-Sr). Also in this study, client-experienced validation correlated .69 with the WAI-Sr. In Bedi and Duff (2014), validation was among the highest rated and most prevalent client-identified alliance formation variables. Validation was also frequently noted as resulting in positive client feelings, which spiraled into increased openness and exploration necessary for alliance formation in the research of Fitzpatrick and colleagues (2006, 2009). The evidence is clear. In the minds of clients, validation is core to developing and maintaining the alliance.

Implications for Practice

It is recommended that clinicians frequently communicate to clients, when possible and appropriate, that they and their thoughts, feelings, and behaviors are acceptable to the clinician, valid, and worthwhile in order to maximize the alliance. Although this construct corresponds greatly with the Rogerian strategy of unconditional positive regard (Rogers, 1961), it is often reported by clients as feeling validated. As a result of this validation, clients should be willing to say things like, "the therapist congratulated me for the things I was doing and had done to help myself" (Bedi, Davis, & Williams, 2005, p. 318) and "the counsellor did not judge me and made me feel like everything I was dealing with was normal" (Simpson & Bedi, 2012, p. 357).

Caveats and Limitations

Similar to any intervention or clinical strategy, clinicians are cautioned to apply the interventions and strategies outlined in this chapter with careful consideration of contextual factors such as unique client characteristics, client preferences, client past experiences, attunement with the client in the moment, timing, clinician skill level, and clinician expertise. For a potentially silly example but one whose underlying principles can be generalized well: the fact that eye contact was noted across research studies as a key clinician behavior that clients strongly believe helped develop and maintain the alliance does not mean that clinicians can just stare incessantly at every client throughout the entire session. There will be times when eye contact should be maintained for longer periods and times when full eye contact should not be made. Timing and appropriateness to the situation are necessary for eye contact to facilitate the development of the alliance.

In addition, there are some notable limitations of the pool of research that this chapter draws on. First, clients' self-report data can be limited by social, cognitive, and memory biases and restrictions (Hyman & Loftus, 1998; Nisbett & Wilson, 1977; Villejoubert, 2005). This includes the notion that there will be variables that impact the working alliance that are beyond the awareness of clients (such as the impact of one's history of positive or negative interpersonal relationships and one's attachment style) (Sharpless, Muran, & Barber, 2010).

Second, despite the massive accumulation of research evidence pertaining to the working alliance, virtually all of it is based on research designs (e.g., correlational, regression, qualitative) that do not justify making cause-and-effect claims. However, there is a growing pool of research and reported clinical experience consistent with claims of causality made in this chapter (e.g., Duff & Bedi, 2010).

Third, most theorizing and research is based on treating alliance and clinical technique as distinct components of treatment. In contrast, Hatcher and Barends (2006) propose that alliance and technique are inseparable—that the alliance is actualized when techniques engage clients in collaborative and purposeful work. So, rather than viewing alliance as a component of the overall therapeutic relationship or as distinct from techniques, Hatcher and Barends (2006) describe the two constructs as necessarily intertwined and requiring each other. According to them, the alliance is what occurs when clinicians' interventions and strategies engage the client toward shared goals and agreed-upon tasks. In other words, the alliance is a result of multiple components of psychological treatment acting together, rather than an isolated component. Techniques that can enhance or embody collaborative purposeful work reflect a sound working alliance (Hatcher & Barends, 2006). Considering alliance and technique as intertwined, while diverging from how the alliance is predominantly understood, actually best embodies the growing body of research on clients' experiences of the working alliance. Adopting this perspective, however, is inconsistent with how the alliance is usually researched.

Fourth, what is offered in this chapter is what clients believe contributes to developing or maintaining the working alliance with their mental health professionals. Extrapolation of these findings to the actual process of alliance formation, which involves interaction between two individuals, should be done cautiously and with consideration for the fact that clients' experiences of the alliance may diverge substantially from clinicians' experiences or personal observations. Clients' subjective experience of establishing a working alliance cannot be equated with, and is therefore not synonymous with the actual interactive process of alliance formation (Duff & Bedi, 2014). In other words, what the client thinks is this one single person's interpretation and understanding of how the alliance is formed and maintained with them, but the alliance is a relationship and requires another person (the clinician) who may see, understand, and experience things differently. Nonetheless, the results within this body of research are suggestive of causal processes to be further investigated in future research.

Summary

Clients' experiences of the alliance are more predictive of therapeutic outcomes than are clinicians' experiences (Flückiger et al., 2018). Growing research on clients' perspectives on, experiences of, and contributions to the working alliance (much of which is qualitative or mixed-methods) seems to counter the dominant understandings of the working alliance, which are based on quantitative research and psychometric measures that are grounded in viewpoints of clinicians (Bedi, 2006). Research privileging the voices of clients has concluded the importance of early interactions in and prior to psychological treatment (Tryon et al., 2007), the relational experience of interventions (Bedi, Davis, & Arvay, 2005; Bedi, Davis, & Williams, 2005), and the value of microskills (MacFarlane et al., 2015) such as validation (Bedi 2006; Bedi, Davis, & Williams, 2005), and has taken a critical look at the lived experience of client collaboration when it comes to developing and maintaining a working alliance (Bedi, 2006). Each of these principles has key practice implications as outlined in this chapter. However, more research is needed on the client perspective for professionals to have a better understanding of how to develop and maintain the working alliance with clients.

References

Anderson, P., Bendtsen, P., Spak, F., Reynolds, J., Drummond, . . . Gual, T. (2016). Improving the delivery of brief interventions for heavy drinking in primary health care: Outcome results of the Optimizing Delivery of Health Care Intervention (ODHIN) five-country cluster randomized factorial trial. *Addiction*, *111*, 1935–1945. doi:10.1111/add.13476

Asay, T. P., & Lambert, M. J. (1999). The empirical case for the common factors in therapy: Quantitative findings. In M. A. Hubble, B. L. Duncan, & S. D. Miller (Eds.), *The heart and soul of change: What works in therapy* (pp. 23–55). Washington, DC: American Psychological Association.

Bachelor, A. (1995). Clients' perception of the therapeutic alliance: A qualitative analysis. *Journal of Counseling Psychology*, *42*, 323–337. doi:10.1037/0022-0167.42.3.323

Barros, P., Altimir, C., & Perez, C. (2016). Patients' facial-affective regulation during episodes of rupture of the therapeutic alliance. *Studies in Psychology*, *37*, 580–603. doi:10.1080/02109395.2016.1204781

Bedi, R. P. (2006). Concept mapping the client's perspective on counseling alliance formation. *Journal of Counseling Psychology*, *53*, 26–35. doi:10.1037/0022-0167.53.1.26

Bedi, R. P., Cook, M. C., & Domene, J. F. (2012). The university student perspective on factors that hinder the counseling alliance. *College Student Journal, 46*, 350–361.

Bedi, R. P., Davis, M. D., & Arvay, M. J. (2005). The client's perspective on forming a counselling alliance and implications for research on counsellor training. *Canadian Journal of Counselling, 39*, 71–85.

Bedi, R. P., Davis, M. D., & Williams, M. (2005). Critical incidents in the formation of the therapeutic alliance from the client's perspective. *Psychotherapy: Theory, Research, Practice, Training, 42*, 311–323. doi:10.1037/0033-3204.42.3.311

Bedi, R. P., & Duff, C. T. (2009). Prevalence of counselling alliance type preferences across two samples. *Canadian Journal of Counselling, 43*, 152.

Bedi, R. P., & Duff, C. T. (2014). Client as expert: A Delphi poll of clients' subjective experience of therapeutic alliance formation variables. *Counselling Psychology Quarterly, 27*, 1–18. doi:10.1080/09515070.2013.857295

Bedi, R. P., & Richards, M. (2011). What a man wants: The male perspective on therapeutic alliance formation. *Psychotherapy, 48*, 381–390. doi:10.1037/a0022424

Benton, J. M., & Overtree, C. E. (2012). Multicultural office design: A case example. *Professional Psychology: Research & Practice, 43*, 265–269. doi:10.1037/a0027443

Blanchard, M., & Farber, B. A. (2016). Lying in psychotherapy: Why and what clients don't tell their therapist about therapy and their relationship. *Counselling Psychology Quarterly, 29*, 90–112. doi:10.1080/09515070.2015.1085365

Bordin, E. S. (1979). The generalizability of the psychoanalytic concept of the working alliance. *Psychotherapy: Theory, Research & Practice, 16*, 252–260. doi:10.1037/h0085885

Borenstein, L. (2006). The therapist's office. *Smith College Studies in Social Work, 76*, 25–37. doi:10.1300/J497v76n03_03

Coutinho, J., Ribeiro, E., Hill, C., & Safran, J. (2011). Therapists' and clients' experiences of alliance ruptures: A qualitative study. *Psychotherapy Research, 21*, 525–540. doi:10.1080/10503307.2011.587469

Crits-Christoph, P., Gibbons, M. B. C., Hamilton, J., Ring-Kurtz, S., & Gallop, R. (2011). The dependability of alliance assessments: The alliance-outcome correlation is larger than you might think. *Journal of Consulting and Clinical Psychology, 79*, 267–278. doi:10.1037/a0023668

Crits-Christoph, P., Gibbons, M. B. C., & Hearon, B. (2006). Does the alliance cause good outcome? Recommendations for future research on the alliance. *Psychotherapy: Theory, Research, Practice, Training, 43*, 280–285. doi:10.1037/0033-3204.43.3.280

Cummings, A. L., Martin, J., Hallberg, E., & Slemon, A. (1992). Memory for therapeutic events, session effectiveness, and working alliance in short-term counseling. *Journal of Counseling Psychology, 39*, 306–312. doi:10.1037/0022-0167.39.3.306

Daniels, T., & Ivey, A. E. (2007). *Microcounseling: Making skills training work in a multicultural world.* Springfield, IL: Charles C. Thomas.

Devlin, A. S., Donovan, S., Nicolov, A., Nold, O., Packard, A., & Zandan, G. (2009). "Impressive?" credentials, family photographs, and the perception of therapist qualities. *Journal of Environmental Psychology, 29*, 503–512. doi:10.1016/j.jenvp.2009.08.008

Devlin, A. S., & Nasar, J. L. (2012). Impressions of psychotherapists' offices: Do therapists and clients agree? *Professional Psychology: Research and Practice, 43*, 118–122. doi:10.1037/a0027292

Duff, C. T., & Bedi, R. P. (2010). Counsellor behaviours that predict therapeutic alliance: From the client's perspective. *Counselling Psychology Quarterly, 23*, 91–110. doi:10.1080/09515071003688165

Duncan, B. L., Miller, S. D., Sparks, J. A., Claud, D. A., Reynolds, L. R., Brown, J., & Johnson, L. D. (2003). The session rating scale: Preliminary psychometric properties of a "working" alliance measure. *Journal of Brief Therapy, 3,* 3–12.

Eames, V., & Roth, A. (2000). Patient attachment orientation and the early working alliance: A study of patient and therapist reports of alliance quality and ruptures. *Psychotherapy Research 10,* 421–434. doi:10.1093/ptr/10.4.421

Elliott, R., & James, E. (1989). Varieties of client experience in psychotherapy: An analysis of the literature. *Clinical Psychology Review, 9,* 443–467. doi:10.1016/0272-7358(89)90003-2

Fitzpatrick, M. R., Janzen, J., Chamodraka, M., Gamberg, S., & Blake, E. (2009). Client relationship incidents in early therapy: Doorways to collaborative engagement. *Psychotherapy Research, 19,* 654–665. doi:10.1080/10503300902878235

Fitzpatrick, M. R., Janzen, J., Chamodraka, M., & Park, J. (2006). Client critical incidents in the process of early alliance development: A positive emotion-exploration spiral. *Psychotherapy Research, 16,* 486–498. doi:10.1080/10503300500485391

Flückiger, C., Del Re, A. C., Wampold, B. E., & Horvath, A. O. (2018). The alliance in adult psychotherapy: A meta-analytic synthesis. *Psychotherapy.* Advance online publication. doi:10.1037/pst0000172

Hartmann, A., Joos, A., Orlinsky, D. E., & Zeeck, A. (2015). Accuracy of therapist perceptions of patients' alliance: Exploring the divergence. *Psychotherapy Research, 25,* 408–419. doi:10.1080/10503307.2014.927601

Hatcher, R. L., & Barends, A. W. (1996). Patients' view of the alliance in psychotherapy: Exploratory factor analysis of three alliance measures. *Journal of Consulting and Clinical Psychology, 64*(6), 1326–1336. doi:10.1037/0022-006X.64.6.1326

Hatcher, R. L., & Barends, A. W. (2006). How a return to theory could help alliance research. *Psychotherapy, 43,* 292–299. doi:10.1037/0033-3204.43.3.292

Hatcher, R. L., Barends, A., Hansell, J., & Gutfreund, M. J. (1995). Patients' and therapists' shared and unique views of the therapeutic alliance: An investigation using confirmatory factor analysis in a nested design. *Journal of Consulting and Clinical Psychology, 63,* 636–643. doi:10.1037/0022-006X.63.4.636

Horvath, A., & Bedi, R. (2002). The alliance. In J. C. Norcross (Ed.), *Psychotherapy relationships that work: Therapist contributions and responsiveness to patients* (pp. 37–69). New York: Oxford University Press.

Hyman, I. E., & Loftus, E. F. (1998). Errors in autobiographical memory. *Clinical Psychology Review, 18,* 933–947. doi:10.1016/S0272-7358(98)00041-5

Kim, E., & Kim, C. (2013). Comparative effects of empathic verbal responses: Reflection versus validation. *Journal of Counseling Psychology, 60,* 439–444. doi:10.1037/a0032786

Kivlighan, D. M. (1990). Relation between counselors' use of interntions and clients' perception of working alliance. *Journal of Counseling Psychology, 37,* 27–32. doi:10.1037//0022-0167.37.1.27

Kivlighan, D. M., Marmarosh, C. L., & Hilsenroth, M. J. (2014). Client and therapist therapeutic alliance, session evaluation, and client reliable change: A moderated actor-partner interdependence model. *Journal of Counseling Psychology, 61,* 15–23. doi:10.1037/a0034939

Kuntze, J., van der Molen, H. T., & Born, M. P. (2009). Increase in counselling communication skills after basic and advanced microskills training. *British Journal of Educational Psychology, 79,* 175–188. doi:10.1348/000709908X313758

Lambert, M. J., Gregersen, A. T., & Burlingame, G. M. (2004). The Outcome Questionnaire-45. In M. E. Maruish (Ed.), *The use of psychological testing for treatment planning and outcomes assessment: Instruments for adults. Volume 3, 3rd ed.* (pp. 191–234). Mahwah, NJ: Lawrence Erlbaum Associates.

Lazarus, A. A. (1993). Tailoring the therapeutic relationship, or being an authentic chameleon. *Psychotherapy: Theory, Research, Practice, Training, 30,* 404–407. doi:10.1037/0033-3204.30.3.404

Levitt, H. M. (2002). The unsaid in the psychotherapy narrative: Voicing the unvoiced. *Counselling Psychology Quarterly, 15,* 333–350. doi:10.1080/0951507021000029667

Lilienfeld, S. O., Ritschel, L. A., Lynn, S. J., Cautin, R. L., & Latzman, R. D. (2014). Why ineffective psychotherapies appear to work: A taxonomy of causes of spurious therapeutic effectiveness. *Perspectives on Psychological Science, 9,* 355–387. doi:10.1177/1745691614535216

Linehan, M. M. (1997). Validation and psychotherapy. In A. Bohart & L. Greenberg (Eds.). *Empathy reconsidered: New directions in psychotherapy* (pp. 353–392). Washington, DC: American Psychological Association.

Luborsky, L. (1976). Helping alliance in psychotherapy. In J. L. Cleghhorn (Ed.), *Successful psychotherapy* (pp. 92–116). New York: Brunner/Mazel.

MacFarlane, P., Anderson, T., & McClintock, A. S. (2015). The early formation of the working alliance from the client's perspective: A qualitative study. *Psychotherapy, 52,* 363–372. doi:10.1037/a0038733

Martin, J., & Stelmaczonek, K. (1988). Participants' identification and recall of important events in counseling. *Journal of Counseling Psychology, 35,* 385–390. doi:10.1037/0022-0167.35.4.385

McLennan, J. (1994). The skills-based model of counselling training: A review of the evidence. *Australian Psychologist, 29,* 79–88. doi:10.1080/00050069408257328

Miller, S. D., Duncan, B. L., Sorrell, R., & Brown, G. S. (2005). The partners for change outcome management system. *Journal of Clinical Psychology, 61,* 199–208. doi:10.1002/jclp.20111

Miya Y., & Hanyu, K. (2006). The effects of interior design on communications and impressions of a counselor in a counseling room. *Environment and Behavior, 38,* 484–502.

Mohr, J. J., & Woodhouse, S. S. (2000, June). Clients' visions of helpful and harmful psychotherapy: An approach to measuring individual differences in therapy priorities. Paper presented at the annual meeting of the Society for Psychotherapy Research, Chicago, Illinois.

Mohr, J. J., & Woodhouse, S. S. (2001). Looking inside the therapeutic alliance: Assessing clients' visions of helpful and harmful psychotherapy. *Psychotherapy Bulletin, 36,* 15–16. doi:10.3389/fpsyg.2011.00270

Muran, J. C., Safran, J. D., Samstag, L. W., & Winston, A. (2005). Evaluating an alliance-focused treatment for personality disorders. *Psychotherapy: Theory, Research, Practice, Training, 42,* 532–545. doi:10.1037/0033-3204.42.4.532

Nasar, J., & Devlin, A. (2011). Impressions of psychotherapists' offices. *Journal of Counseling Psychology, 58,* 310–320. doi:10.1037/a0023887.

Nisbett, R. E., & Wilson, T. D. (1977). Telling more than we know: Verbal reports on mental processes. *Psychological Review 84,* 231–259. doi:10.1037/0033-295X.84.3.231

Norcross, J. C., & Beutler, L. E. (1997). Determining the therapeutic relationship of choice in brief therapy. In J. N. Butcher (Ed.), *Personality assessment in managed health care: A practitioner's guide: Using the MMPI-2 in treatment planning* (pp. 42–60). New York: Oxford University Press.

Puschner, B., Wolf, M., & Kraft, S. (2008). Helping alliance and outcome in psycho-therapy: What predicts what in routine outpatient treatment? *Psychotherapy Research,* *18,* 167–178.

Rennie, D. L. (1994). Storytelling in psychotherapy: The client's subjective experience. *Psychotherapy: Theory, Research, Practice, Training, 31,* 234–243. doi:10.1037/h0090224

Rhodes, R. H., Hill, C. E., Thompson, B. J., & Elliott, R. (1994). Client retrospective re-call of resolved and unresolved misunderstanding events. *Journal of Counseling Psychology, 41,* 473–483. doi:10.1037/0022-0167.41.4.473

Richards, M., & Bedi, R. P. (2015). Gaining perspective: How men describe incidents damaging the therapeutic alliance. *Psychology of Men & Masculinity, 16,* 170–182. doi:10.1037/a0036924

Ridley, C. R., Kelly, S. M., & Mollen, D. (2011). Microskills training: Evolution, reexam-ination, and call for reform. *The Counseling Psychologist, 39,* 800–824. doi:10.1177/0011000010378438

Rogers, C. R. (1961). *On becoming a person.* Oxford: Houghton Mifflin.

Safran, J. D., & Muran, J. C. (2000). Resolving therapeutic alliance ruptures: Diversity and integration. *Journal of Clinical Psychology, 56,* 233–243. doi:10.1002/(SICI)1097-4679(200002)56:2<233::AID-JCLP9>3.0.CO;2-3

Safran, J., Muran, J., & Eubanks-Carter, C. (2011). Repairing alliance ruptures. *Psychotherapy, 48,* 224–238. doi:10.1093/acprof:oso/9780199737208.003.0011.

Sharpless, B. A., Muran, J. C., & Barber, J. P. (2010). Coda: Recommendations for practice and training. In J. C. Muran, & J. P. Barber (Eds.), *The therapeutic alliance: An evidence based-guide to practice* (pp. 338–350). New York: Guilford Press.

Simpson, A. J., & Bedi, R. P. (2012). The therapeutic alliance: Clients' categorization of client-identified factors. *Canadian Journal of Counselling and Psychotherapy, 46,* 344–366.

Smith, J. D., & Agate, J. (2004). Solutions for overconfidence: Evaluation of an instruc-tional module for counselor trainees. *Counselor Education and Supervision, 44,* 31–43. doi:10.1002/j.1556-6978.2004.tb01858.x

Swift, J. K., & Greenberg, R. P. (2015). *Premature termination in psychotherapy: Strategies for engaging clients and improving outcomes.* Washington, DC: APA Books.

Tryon, G. S., Blackwell, S. C., & Hammel, E. F. (2007). A meta-analytic examination of client-therapist perspectives of the working alliance. *Psychotherapy Research, 17,* 629–642. doi:10.1080/10503300701320611

Villejoubert, G. (2005). Could they have known better? Review of the special issue of memory on the hindsight bias. *Applied Cognitive Psychology, 19,* 140–143.

Wampold, B. E. (2001). *The great psychotherapy debate: Models, methods, and findings.* Mahwah, NJ: Lawrence Erlbaum Associates.

Wampold, B. E., & Imel, Z. E. (2015). *The great psychotherapy debate: The evidence for what makes psychotherapy work* (2nd ed.). New York: Routledge.

Wright-McDougal, J. J., & Toriello, P. J. (2013). Ethical implications of confirmation bias in the rehabilitation counseling relationship. *Journal of Applied Rehabilitation Counseling, 44,* 3–10.

Zilcha-Mano, S., Muran, J. C., Hungr, C., Eubanks, C. F., Safran, J. D., & Winston, A. (2016). The relationship between alliance and outcome: Analysis of a two-person per-spective on alliance and session outcome. *Journal of Consulting and Clinical Psychology, 84,* 484–496. doi:10.1037/ccp0000058

7

Multicultural Considerations in the Working Alliance

Changming Duan

As noted by the editor in the first chapter, the working alliance goes beyond therapist–client agreement on goals, tasks, and the formation of a bond and reflects an overarching sense of consensus, collaboration, and shared mission between therapist and clients. The research conducted on the working alliance to date has made an indisputably strong case that the working alliance is a necessary condition of effective therapy, and its importance cannot be overemphasized in obtaining desirable intervention outcomes. In this chapter, I focus on specific aspects of building the working alliance in multicultural therapy relationships.

After serious considerations, I decided to focus on racial and/or ethnic domains of multiculturalism and diversity in this chapter to provide space for concentrated discussion on the topic. However, I want to remind readers that attention to client identity intersectionality (Crenshaw, 1989) is critically important if we are to understand clients holistically and accurately. No clients are from cultural backgrounds that are limited to one dimension, such as race or ethnicity, but contain multiple identifications in gender, socioeconomic status (SES), sexual orientation, and so on. Their experience of life can only be understood in their cultural contexts, which are determined by how they are treated by others and society as well as their own values and worldviews. Focused discussion of race- and ethnicity-related issues in relation to the working alliance is of great importance and utility because it is one visible and salient aspect of an individual's identity, and these issues are closely associated with their experience of privilege/oppression in society (Page & Shepherd, 2010). I do hope that some of the content discussed here will stimulate readers to think about its relevance to their work with clients who represent the broader scope of human diversity, including gender, sexual orientation, social class, religion, physical disability, and more.

Race is a socially constructed construct, not a biological one, and it is linked to "a very powerful social reality" (Altman, 2007, p. 15). Society uses race to classify individuals with different physical features (e.g., skin color) and other schemes (e.g., tribal affiliations, nationalities, languages, etc.); thus, individuals' biological features are associated with their social experience in terms of how they are treated by others at individual and institutional levels. With both similar and different connotations, ethnicity is viewed as a broad concept referring to individuals' cultural characteristics in terms of values, beliefs, and behaviors (Betancourt & Lopez, 1993). In the psychological literature, it is often interchangeably used with race and viewed mostly as involving beliefs, norms, behaviors, language, and intuitions (Hays, 2016) among non-Caucasian groups such as Asian American, Native American, or Mexican American. In this chapter, these two terms are used together and/or interchangeably to refer to non-Caucasian individuals and sometimes the term "people of color" is also used.

As expected, racial/ethnic identity has been observed as being associated with various self-related (e.g., self-esteem, academic achievement, and mental health or stress, depression and physical health conditions) and other-focused (e.g., trust or mistrust of others, ingroup and outgroup attitudes, perception of the working alliance, and satisfaction about counseling) psychological experiences for minority group members. In therapeutic contexts, racial/ethnic minority clients have been found to face greater challenges than whites in forming trusting working alliances with therapists due to perceived or actual cultural differences and/or cultural biases and discrimination (Smith & Trimble, 2016). Thus, it is worthwhile discussing ways in which this phenomenon can be corrected to create therapeutic environments in which racial and ethnic minority clients enjoy a good working alliance with their therapists and experience therapy as facilitative and helpful.

Other chapters in this volume provide theoretical support and practical guides in terms of how therapists pursue the working alliance with clients by strengthening the working bond and setting agreed-upon goals and tasks. This chapter's focus will discuss what therapists can do in this pursuit when working with ethnic/racial minority clients. Although this task may be most challenging for white therapists, therapists of color are not exempt from the challenge. Even when sharing clients' racial and ethnic minority status, therapists still need to make deliberate efforts to overcome the influence of their biased training and knowledge biases (e.g., by theories built for the mainstream culture), other social statuses (e.g., as trained therapists), and differences in other contextual areas. It is absolutely the therapist's responsibility and obligation to forge and strengthen the therapist–client working alliance with the goal of helping the clients. Failure to do so may lead to harm to clients, particularly to those clients from minority groups that are already marginalized by society.

In this discussion of how to improve therapist competency in building the working alliance with racial and ethnic minority clients, I made the following assumptions based on accumulated research evidence and clinical observations: (1) the working alliance is the most critical and powerful condition for effective therapy, *especially* when working with minority clients; (2) therapist, client, and context all play a role in the development of the working alliance, and therapists have the major responsibility to work toward an optimal working alliance with all clients and in all client contexts; (3) therapist respect for and appreciation of individual and cultural diversity, as well as understanding of the system of social privilege and oppression, are critical conditions for building and maintaining the working alliance with the culturally diverse and socially marginalized; (4) many of the challenges in developing and sustaining the working alliance exist regardless of therapists' racial and ethnic backgrounds; and (5) failure to achieve a healthy working alliance with ethnic and racial minority clients leads to limited clinical outcomes and possibly even harm. With these assumptions, we can see some general directions and areas of learning for those therapists who are interested in and committed to improving their ability and skills in forming strong working alliances with racial minority clients.

Therapist "Being" as the Basis for "Doing": Needed Self-Work for the Purpose of Helping

One unique feature of the psychotherapy profession is that the most important tools therapists have in helping clients are themselves, and therapists' "being" is relevant and intimately related to their doing. In fact, the personal being is the foundation for a therapist's professional therapeutic competence. As Carl Rogers's notion of therapist genuineness being a facilitative condition implies, therapist being plays an important role in clients' experience of therapy. In his words in *A Way of Being* (1980), Rogers stated that "The more the therapist is him or herself in the relationship, putting up no professional front or façade, the greater is the likelihood that the client will change and grow in a constructive manner" (p. 115). He also shared, in his reflection of his theory of personal development, that "It is that the individual has within himself or herself vast resources for self-understanding, for altering his or her self-concept, attitudes and self-directed behavior—and that these resources can be tapped if only a definable climate of facilitative psychological attitudes can be provided" (Rogers, 1986, p. 258). Therapist "being" (i.e., accepting, genuine, congruent, and empathic) is necessary for creating facilitative attitudes and conditions for clients. When entering a therapeutic relationship, minority clients need to feel safe, accepted, and respected, which is sometimes missing in their social experience.

Research has shown that therapist factors contribute significantly to psychotherapy outcome (e.g., Wampold & Brown, 2005), meaning that some therapists are more or less effective than others (e.g., Kraus, Castonguay, Boswell, Nordberg, & Hayes, 2011), and therapist qualities matter in their ability to build a working alliance (Castonguay & Hill, 2017; Strupp, 1998). As revealed by a comprehensive review of empirical studies on the working alliance by Horvath and Bedi (2002), a therapist being warm, accepting, engaged, empathic, and responsive is facilitative of the alliance. A therapist being open, flexible, and respectful was also highly correlated with ratings of the working alliance (Ackerman & Hilsenroth, 2001, 2003). Through a series of studies, Heinonen (2014) demonstrated that therapists' professional and personal characteristics play an important role in the formation of the working alliance with clients, including a therapist being professionally confident and interpersonally active, with an engaging manner and a deliberate, nonintrusive, and considerate relational stance.

On the other hand, however, therapist lack of enjoyment or engagement while seeing clients was found to negatively predict the working alliance (Heinonen, 2014), and those therapists who showed a "take-charge" attitude early in therapy (Lichenberg et al., 1988), irritability toward clients (Sexton, 1996), and being perceived as "cold" (Hersoug, Monsen, Havik, & Hogland, 2000) tend to face poor or deteriorating alliances. Therapist being rigid, tense, or inattentive, and inappropriately using self-disclosures or insisting on using interpretation that is not needed or appropriate also negatively influenced the alliance (Ackerman & Hilsenroth, 2001, 2003). Similarly, a study by Nissen-Lie, Monsen, and Ronnestad (2010) revealed that therapists' experience of negative reactions to clients and therapists' self-doubt contributed to clients' experience of stress in the therapeutic relationship. These findings offer unequivocal support to the importance of therapist being and the need for therapists to continuously work on themselves toward becoming open, flexible, attentive, engaged, and confident. There are unique challenges for therapists to develop and display these qualities of being toward clients whose racial, ethnical, and cultural backgrounds are diverse and if their backgrounds have been historically marginalized. In addition to unfamiliarity or "not knowing," internalization of the prejudice, biases, and discrimination prevalent in society post challenges for therapists' self-work in this area.

Becoming a person with optimal personal qualities for helping others is probably the result of socialization, development, and learning, which occur in contexts and reflect one's culture and experience as well as predispositions. It is not so difficult to see that—due to individuals' general and relative lack of contact with people who are different from them in life and due to the fact that society awards privilege and social power differentially according to people's demographics—therapists' socialization may not have equipped them with the readiness to relate and respond to individuals of different racial and ethnic backgrounds as much as to people from their familiar groups. The research on individuals' affective reactions to ingroup and outgroup members (e.g., Brown, Bradley, & Lang, 2006) supports the expectation that therapists may generally find it more difficult to naturally show warmth, openness, confidence, engagement, and many other good qualities of being to those whose social positions are different due to their being persons of color. The deliberate effort in a personal and professional journey toward being multiculturally competent and social justice–oriented is needed for therapists to effectively connect with culturally diverse clients and build trusting therapeutic alliances. In other words, developing the self is the therapist's responsibility and the basis for effective work in building and strengthening the working alliance with diverse clients. One of the oldest adages in psychotherapy remains true to this day and is particularly relevant to this chapter: "Therapist know thyself" and, particularly important is "know thyself in relation to others."

For responsible and conscientious therapists, continuously and persistently doing the self-work to nurture facilitative attitudes and characteristics toward culturally and socially diverse clients is a way of being. It involves the therapist's willingness to challenge existing biases and prejudices and adopt a new worldview that is inclusive and respectful of racial, ethnic, and cultural diversity. They need to be able to genuinely *feel* the respect for and appreciation of those who are different from themselves in race, ethnicity, social status, and/or worldviews and values so that they can show genuine warmth, acceptance, appreciation, enjoyment, and attentiveness when working with them. The working alliance implies therapists being allies with their clients, being with them on a shared mission, and being on the same page with the client as far as the work in therapy is concerned. To do this more effectively with a diverse clientele, therapist can consider the following personal psychological work and preparation:

1. *Understanding the multicultural self.* To understand clients with different cultural backgrounds, therapists need to be in touch with the cultural aspects of themselves. In a diverse society, everyone is multicultural in the sense that their experiences of life are related to who they are demographically. Some people may have the privilege of not seeing themselves as being multicultural because their race or ethnicity has not brought them unearned oppression/disadvantage; they have always fit with the power groups. However, it should be noted that there are always others paying for their privilege and suffering from their unawareness of cultural diversity because, in interpersonal interactions, individuals consciously or unconsciously contribute to each other's sense of self, social position, and relationships (Duan & Brown, 2015). For example, a white person's "I do

not see color" attitude may make him or her feel "fair" while making a person of color feel unsafe. In psychotherapy settings, a white therapist may show his being moral and just by promoting meritocracy, but his honored "pull up the bootstraps" strategy may hurt the working alliance with clients of color. Thus, responsible therapists account for their race and ethnicity and intentionally learn about their own cultures, the relationship between their culture and other cultures, and the ways in which they enjoy privileges that others have not solely on the basis of race and ethnicity. Pondering on questions such as what being a Caucasian (or African, Asian, Latino, Native) American means in this society and for oneself, or what one's being Caucasian (or African, Asian, Latino, Native) means to others may help us gain awareness of our own biases, prejudices, or lack of understanding of the culturally diverse. This work may cultivate the therapist's ability to engage with and show acceptance and empathy to diverse clients.

2. *Being informed of current social, cultural, and political issues in the public and trying to understand their impact on racial/ethnic minorities.* To increase the readiness to respond, respect, and empathize with ethnic minority clients requires therapists to be aware of clients' contextual experience. Whether or not therapists are interested, public events surely influence their diverse clients' psychological experience. For instance, the Black Lives Matter movement burst onto the national scene in 2016 as a protest against violence toward African Americans. If therapists are informed of it and have reflected on its meaning and influence, they may be more able to see their own roles in it and more readily support African American clients to navigate their perceptions and experience to reach psychological benefit. Being sensitive to and mindful of their diverse clients' social and cultural contexts is a good quality that therapists can intentionally nurture within themselves, one that will facilitate their ability to be "allies" with their clients in therapy.

3. *Training our brain to reduce implicit biases. Implicit bias* refers to "the unconscious and unintentional assumptions people make about each other" (Gonzalez et al., 2018, p. 1669) and has been found to negatively impact racial/ethnic disparity in healthcare and patients' experience of clinical encounters (e.g., Blair et al., 2013). For instance, research has shown that, unintentionally, doctors were less likely to recommend cardiac catheterization (a helpful procedure) to black patients—even when their medical files were statistically identical to those of white patients (Jacobson, 2015). A black-sounding name makes people imagine a larger, more dangerous, and lower SES person than a character with a white-sounding name (Holbrook, Fessler, & Navarrete, 2016). Such implicit biases are probably

present more than we want to believe and may influence therapist clinical decision-making. Thus, in order to be prepared for building the working alliance with ethnic minority clients, responsible therapists may take on the challenge of reducing implicit bias. To make progress in this difficult task, we may need to first acknowledge that we do have implicit biases about racial minorities and recognize our vulnerable areas before doing deliberate practice or intentional correction. One way to become aware is to use available tests such as the Harvard Implicit Association Test (IAT), which is available online https://www.glaxdiversitycouncil.com/resources/harvard-implicit-association-test-iat/. This test allows each of us to discover our unconscious and covert biases toward minority clients.

In terms of strategies to undo unconscious stereotypes and biases toward racial/ethnic minorities, intentional and deliberative effort is needed to find ways that fit our individual situations. It may be that some of the methods that Tropp and Godsil (2015) outlined can be effective for some of us. Their suggestions include exposing ourselves to counterstereotypic examples of minority groups (e.g., intentionally learning about the life of ethnic minority leaders, about energetic Native Americans, or about unassuming yet self-confident black women); consciously contrasting negative stereotypes with specific counterexamples (e.g., when hearing "Latino men are all macho," consciously think about all Latino men that you know or are positive figures in the public); seeking specific information about members of specific racial groups rather than being color-blind (e.g., reading a theory by a minority scholar, learning about his or her life story as a member of the minority group); assuming the perspective of an outgroup member (e.g., before reacting to a news report about an incident in which a white police officer shot a black unarmed man, trying to put yourself in the shoes of a black person in front of this event); and generating positive interactions with members of racial minority groups (e.g., nurturing good working relationships with minority colleagues at work). We can integrate these tactics into our daily life, such as being thoughtful about what movies we watch, how we process news of current events, trying to take the perspectives of "others" whenever possible, and being on guard for our hypothesis-confirming tendency in relation to race, ethnicity, and culture. Dr. Mahzarin Banaji (2018), one of the major scholars of implicit bias theories, shared one very inspiring and moving strategy in a Public Radio Interview program. She said that in order to eliminate her implicit bias toward Middle Eastern Islamic group after the 9/11 tragedy, she used diverse people's faces including diverse Middle Easterners as her computer screen saver. In this way, she trained her brain not to react stereotypically when seeing individuals from different cultures.

Diverse Social Realities: Understanding Implications of the System of Oppression and Privilege

Not everyone living in the United States is in the same social reality. In addition to individual differences related to psychological health, there is pain and inequality from social oppression in the life of the racial/ethnic minorities in a society where the privileged dominate (Brown et al., 2000). As stated by diversity and social justice trainer and consultant Diane Goodman (2015), "One way to define oppression is as a system of advantage (privilege) and disadvantage (oppression) based on social group membership. Some groups are advantaged—seen as superior, have greater social power, and receive unearned benefits, while other groups are disadvantaged—seen as inferior, have less social power and face discrimination and violence" (p. 2). This system has created an uneven distribution of power, and it has led to gross racial and ethnic disparities in many areas of life, including in economics, education, employment, health, and healthcare (Duan & Brown, 2015). As reported by a work group of the American Psychological Association, racial and ethnic minorities in the United States consistently reported having greater exposure to discrimination, higher levels of stress, and having to endure a lot more negative, aversive, and even denigrating conditions than members of the majority group (Brondolo et al., 2017).

A full discussion of the system of oppression and privilege is beyond the scope of this chapter, but it is important that therapists understand its implications and relevance in our work with ethnic minority clients. In counseling rooms, this system is often present, whether or not we invite it in. Therapists and clients unavoidably bring with them their respective experienced social reality to the therapeutic relationship, in which client presenting concerns and therapeutic experience interact with the social realities and cultural identities of both parties. Thus, to effectively build a working alliance with clients who are influenced by this system, therapists' understanding of *their* experienced context is extremely important. For instance, the knowledge that some African American men growing up in poor inner-city neighborhoods are socialized to be wary of white people in order to protect themselves (see Coates, 2015) may help a white therapist to appreciate an African American client's psychology, including possibly the lack of trust or the ambivalence that they bring into therapy. The understanding that the therapist being white means something more than an individual self-identifier may prompt the therapist to attend to how minority clients' experiences have contributed to their clinical symptoms. Furthermore, being able to acknowledge that some members of our society are unfairly discriminated against on the basis of race or ethnicity may allow therapists to properly evaluate client symptoms in a broader context. This fuller understanding may be an important contributor to building a working alliance with clients of color.

Let's see an example of a white therapist attempting to connect with an African American man mandated by the local police to come to counseling.

THERAPIST: I am glad you are here. Use your own words and tell me why you are here and how I can help you.

CLIENT: I do not know. Don't ask me!

THERAPIST: I want to be helpful to you.

CLIENT: I am not a child. I don't need your help, don't try to fool me!

THERAPIST: You do not sound happy to be here.

CLIENT: Don't try to fool me doc, I'm not stupid!

THERAPIST: It seems that you remember being fooled before.

CLIENT: Yah! You tell me!

THERAPIST: I guess looking at me reminds you of that because I represent people who have fooled you in the past.

CLIENT: Well . . . I don't know. Don't know.

THERAPIST: You know how to protect yourself, and I don't blame you. You are doing it right now, effectively, protecting yourself from someone who reminds you of the bad experience or when you do not feel safe.

CLIENT: I didn't feel unsafe, you know. Just, just that, when I am out of my neighborhood, I am scared. I have no control.

THERAPIST: I really appreciate your sensitivity to the environment and not wanting to put yourself at risk when you are out of your safe zone.

CLIENT: I just, just don't want to be, you know, be so helpless and powerless.

THERAPIST: Give me a chance, actually give *us* a chance, to create a safety zone for you right here, what do you say?

CLIENT: Maybe it won't hurt to try.

This example shows that by acknowledging previously hurtful and demeaning experiences with power groups in the past, the therapist was able to turn attention to the client's social experiences and reasons behind his uncooperative behavior. To build a therapeutic bond with minority clients, such an effort may be worthwhile and necessary, and earning client trust in itself is therapeutic, even if it did not address the problem directly.

When working with clients of color, therapists face the negative impact of the system of privilege and oppression, which has compromised society's mental health delivery system (Smedley, Stith, & Nelson, 2003). Ethnic minorities often have less access to quality care (McGuire & Miranda, 2008), and, when they do receive care, "it is more likely to be of poorer quality" (Bussing & Gray, 2012, p. 663). As noted by Sue (2003), among those who have received care, "rather than feeling that they have been provided benefits, clients often feel invalidated, abused, misunderstood, and oppressed by their providers" (p. 5). This racial/ethnic disparity in mental health was noted by the supplement to the Report by the United States Surgeon General in 2001 (Satcher, 2001), and, 16 years later, the American Psychological Association (APA, 2016) reported that people of color within the United States are still underserved and inadequately served in mental health.

This system has also influenced mental health practice as well. For instance, a tendency has been documented toward ethnic minority clients receiving more misdiagnoses and/or overdiagnoses for psychotic disorders than their white counterparts (Schwartz & Blankenship, 2014). Using the database of Veterans Affairs (VA) system, an examination of 134,523 veterans' diagnosis revealed that race is the most significant demographic variable associated the diagnosis of schizophrenia, with 4.05 and 3.15 more likelihood for African American and Hispanics than for Euro-American veterans (Blow et al., 2004). A review of 24 years of empirical literature (Schwartz & Blankenship, 2014) also uncovered "a clear and pervasive pattern" (p. 133) that psychotic disorder diagnosis was assigned to African American/black clients three to four times more often.

Researchers have attributed this overdiagnosis to racism and a lack of trust in ethnic minority clients' responses to queries about their symptoms. This was described as diagnosis on the basis of "a suspicion of symptoms denial, poor insight, or uncooperativeness" (Goldman, 2012, p. 847). Relatedly, Blow et al. (2004) identified provider biases as one possible explanation because "race appears to matter and still appears to adversely pervade the clinical encounter, whether consciously or otherwise" (p. 846). Misdiagnosing and/or overdiagnosing are examples of assigning a mental disorder diagnosis primarily based on personal prejudices and/or stereotypes about racial/ethnic minority clients, a wrong-doing by "good-willed" clinicians who probably unintentionally brought the system of bias/oppression into psychological services.

Regardless of therapists' race/ethnicity, it takes deliberate effort to learn, reflect, and practice in order to be able to understand the role of racism and oppression in clients' lives and to translate this understanding into therapeutic understanding and interactions to strengthen the working alliance. *To learn*, therapists may develop interest in the life experiences and perspectives of ethnic minorities. Implied in the concept of experiential learning, responsible therapists may choose to attend events that expose them to diverse people, read books or watch movies that reflect minority people's life and perspectives, and keep up with the professional literature that addresses diversity issues. *To reflect*, therapists can explore how they themselves have been socialized and reinforced for seeing the world the way they do and how their view of others may differ from how others see themselves and the world. Most importantly, therapists reflect on the meaning of their social positions to gain awareness about the roles their cultural identities play in the lives of ethnic minority clients. *To practice*, therapists may intentionally train themselves to see what is right among the "wrongs" and what is hidden among the obvious in cross-cultural and social settings, thus cultivating a willingness to stay open and offer others the "benefit of doubt." These exercises may help therapists increase their ability to establish and maintaining working alliances because accurate understanding of clients in their social context is a condition for psychological connections with them.

Pursuing Bond, Collaborative Goals, and Tasks in Therapy: Facilitative Conditions, Skills, and Practices

Working alliance research has produced robust and convincing evidence that having a strong and healthy bond with collaborative goals and tasks is a positive indicator of both the process and outcome of therapy (see Martin, Garske, & Davis, 2000). After a comprehensive review, Hatcher and Barends (2006) concluded that the "Alliance is actualized in therapist techniques, client participation, and the dyad's relational features. Alliance is a property of all components of therapy, a concept superordinate to these components and not a component itself" (p. 292). Psychotherapy often means doing difficult work, and working with ethnic minorities may involve additional challenges due to the fact that the therapist and client may live in different social realities. However, deliberate practice rooted in cultural understanding and respect will help.

Using the guiding questions raised by Hatcher and Barends, " 'Do you like and respect your therapist enough to do the work you expect to do in therapy?' and 'Does your therapist respect and appreciate you enough to permit you to work effectively in therapy' " (p. 296), I discuss several foci that therapists may consider adopting when working with the culturally diverse. The overarching theme of these foci is that therapists prioritize and emphasize working alliance building, not fixating on problems or reducing symptoms, and that they allow the alliance to be "actualized in therapist techniques, client participation, and the dyad's relational features" (p. 292). Therapists have a significant role to play to facilitate the formation of the working alliance by showing respect for and earning respect from clients through therapeutic interactions, which may be more demanding of the therapist when working in a cross-racial therapeutic relationship.

Attending to Client Views and Perspectives

Perspective-taking—viewing the world from the client's perspective—is a major expression of intellectual empathy and a critical contributor to the working alliance (Duan & Sager, 2018). However, we know that often therapists' views differ from those of clients, at least concerning their experience of therapy outcomes, be it session evaluation (Stiles, 2002), therapy effectiveness (Greenberg, 1986), working alliance (Fitzpatrick, Iwakabe, & Stalikas, 2005), or reasons to leave therapy (Gager, 2004). We also know that "only client ratings of the alliance were significantly correlated with positive session impacts" (Fitzpatrick, Iwakabe, & Stalikas, 2005, p. 69) and that "the patient's assessment predicts the outcome of psychotherapy" (Castonguay, Constantino, & Holtforth, 2006). This observation may not be too difficult for us to understand, but it should alarm us, and it calls for heightened attention to how our clients perceive and experience us as therapists in therapeutic relationships, as well as in their world of life. Standing in our own shoes and using our theories and familiar tools, we may not truly understand our clients and, worse yet, may not even know when we failed to understand them.

Let's consider the following clinical vignette.

Tingli is a 52-year-old Asian American female who emigrated from Taiwan with her parents when she was 8 years old. She has a master's degree in computer science and worked for a high-technology company. She sought counseling from a white, middle-aged, experienced female counselor (Dr. D.) after having "bad fights" with her husband. Her husband is also a successful information technology professional working with a large company. They and their teenage daughter live in a middle to upper scale neighborhood that is heavily occupied by Asian Americans in the high-tech professions in a large city. Here are some verbal exchanges she has with the therapist in the first session:

DR. D: My front office assistant told me that you have had conflicts with your husband. Can you tell me in your own words what are your concerns and how I can help you?

TINGLI: [Silence.]

DR. D: Maybe it will be easier, just tell me what had happened between you and your husband that led you here?

TINGLI: We had a fight, a bad one last week, and we do not know what to do. Our daughter was unhappy and went to stay with a friend. [Silence.] It has been 3 days now. What should I do?

DR. D: Sounds like this fight was really bad. Can you say more about it?

TINGLI: We do not like to fight, and we seldom fight. This is bad.

DR. D: I can see that. What did your husband do to you, and how are you feeling about it?

TINGLI: We just fought. I was not able to control myself. My daughter was
angry. He was not pushing her, but I fell on her.
DR. D: Sounds like your husband was violent.
TINGLI: Oh No! Uhmmm, I don't know. Uhmmm, maybe. But [silent]. No.

We can see a possible direction Dr. D. may take after this interaction—focusing
on the husband, husband–wife relationship, how to repair or leave the broken
relationship, and so on. This direction is probably a familiar and common one,
and it may be helpful to many clients. However, if we consider Tingli's culture
and social context, we may want to work harder in understanding and respecting
her perspective. Any or all of these possibilities may exist: her daughter is her
major concern, she does not feel she needed help with her relationship with her
husband, the risk of discussing her negative emotion toward her husband is too
high because she loves him and wants to have harmony, or she is afraid of the
potential consequences if others (in the Asian American community) know her
situation. Thus, therapists may want to focus on understanding the client's perspective and not to see her unwillingness to go into certain directions as resistance or unwillingness to share. To establish a therapeutic bond, it does not help
that Dr. D jumped onto the perceived problems and neglected the client's perspective. Dr. D may want to focus more on supporting Tingli emotionally and
learning about her most pressing needs at this time, her views of her experienced
conflict, and her specific concerns about her daughter and about her marital relationship. Being seen as a problem or a source of the problem (vs. as a person
with emotions and concerns) may discourage some Asian clients from forming a
therapeutic bond with their therapists.

Being Culturally Humble
One relatively recent line of thinking and research focuses on promoting therapist cultural humility in connecting and working with clients whose cultural
identity, values, and worldviews are different from their therapists'. *Cultural
humility* is referred to as the therapist's "ability to maintain an interpersonal
stance that is other-oriented (or open to the other) in relation to aspects of cultural identity that are most important to the client . . . therapists who are more
culturally humble approach clients with respectful openness and work collaboratively with clients to understand the unique intersections of clients' various
aspects of identities and how that affects the developing therapy alliance" (Hook,
Davis, Owen, Worthington, & Utsey, 2013, p. 354). Cultural humility allows
therapists to effectively reduce social distance and share power with the powerless and show respect to clients who have been socially neglected or marginalized
(Ramanathan, 2014). In a study of client perceptions of psychotherapy, Owen

et al. (2016) discovered that therapist cultural humility facilitates the therapeutic relationship with ethnic minority clients and is positively correlated with client improvement.

How to cultivate and communicate therapist cultural humility to clients is one area that deserves attention in the effort of facilitating the working alliance. First, culturally humble healthcare providers share some characteristics, according to Tervalon and Murray-Garcia (1998).

1. *Incorporating a lifelong process of commitment to self-evaluation and self-critique in terms of cultural assumptions and biases.* Unlearning biased and prejudicial views that resulted from one's cultural socialization is not easy. For instance, the myth of meritocracy has deep roots in our belief system, and we need critical self-examination to recognize its potential for harming people of color (Godfrey, Santos, & Burson, 2017). This learning is a life-long process and needs to occur repeatedly in our interaction with minority clients.

2. *Redressing the power imbalances in society through the therapist–client dynamic.* For instance, when the therapist represents the oppressor in any dimension of human diversity, client experience of the therapeutic relationship is influenced by the power dynamic with the therapist that is familiar to them in society. The therapist has the opportunity to redress this imbalance, and failure to do so may compromise the working alliance with the client;.

3. *Developing nonpaternalistic clinical and advocacy partnerships with communities and clients.* Therapists may influence clients' mental health and therapeutic experiences through relating to and joining in with clients and their communities. Working with them, not for them, in promoting health and healthy environments requires therapist involvement in advocacy for racial/ethnic parity at the community and societal levels as well as at the individual level.

Second, these characteristics can be translated into a number of other-focused, respectful, and relationship-oriented stances that bring the culture, cultural identity, and cultural experiences of both clients and therapists into therapeutic relationships. Here are some examples of cultural humility–led actions:

1. *Therapists openly acknowledge racial and/or cultural differences that exist between them and their clients, recognizing their own knowledge gap about the client culture and openly affirming their commitment to being open and collaborating with clients to understand them in their contexts.* For instance, during the initial sessions with a client of color, a white therapist may

consider saying something like "Thank you for being here. Before we start I want to acknowledge some areas of difference between us. I know that this may or may not be directly related to the reason you are here today, but I am aware that being a white person, I have not experienced the world and society in the same way you have, and my views may have been biased by my experience. My promise to you is that I will learn with you during our work together and be helpful to you. I do need your help. If at any time you feel that what I say does not feel right to you or I misunderstand you or your experience, I would be really appreciative if you can tell me."

2. *Therapists recognize contextual reasons and triggers for client symptoms among ethnic minorities, which may result in a reduced risk to pathologize culture- or context-driven behaviors.* For instance, knowing how inner-city African American youth experience the police force, we would not automatically assume that their anger and even destructive behaviors reflects antisocial personality; recognizing how Native Americans may feel being stripped of their indigenous national identity as well as their land and resources, we would not evaluate certain behaviors, such as drinking behavior, as a disease of addiction; understanding, how relationship dominates some Asian communities and individuals, we would not view their inability to stand up to their parents, their bosses, or even their equals as reflecting a weak ego; and understanding how Latina women view their roles in the family, we could avoid automatic association between their lack of self-confidence with negative mental health. In theory, few psychotherapists would deny the fact that racism, oppression, and marginalization are real and influence ethnic minorities' life and social experience, but integrating this understanding into the therapy process requires intentional effort. Being culturally humble means adopting a willingness to question personal assumptions and becoming interested in seeing the possible deleterious effects of racism and oppression on mental health. Perhaps therapists can adopt a mindset that prompts them to always ask these questions: What are the possibilities that this client's difficulties are reflective of the negative effects of racism? What are my assumptions about this client's symptom (e.g., anxiety) and its etiology? In what ways is this very expression of anxiety telling a story of someone being unfairly treated? How might the client be manifesting an array of negative social experiences via his or her symptoms?

3. *Therapists take responsibility when a therapy session is not going smoothly.* For instance, there are times when difficulties occur in therapist–client relationships, such as tensions and raptures in the relationship, the client disagreeing with the therapist on needed tasks, or therapists deeming client goals as unproductive. Research has shown that the therapist's ability or

style of responding matters in such challenging situations. Therapists who respond in an open and nondefensive manner and take responsibility for the problem tend to receive higher ratings of client-reported working alliance (Nissen-Lie, Monsen, & Ronnestad, 2010). We can reason that therapist cultural humbleness and sensitivity may provide a corrective experience for clients who probably have experienced powerful people as being generally unapologetic and other-blaming in society. We see the power of therapist humbleness in earning client cooperation and trust in the following case example.

Juan is a 22-year-old black man who is a single Haitian immigrant. He was brought into a community mental health clinic for treatment for anxiety by his mother. Juan has had two sessions with a female Asian American therapist. During the third session, Juan shut down and barely said anything during the second half of the session, and he left without scheduling for the following week. Through supervision, the therapist became aware that Juan became stressed and quiet after she started inquiring about his hallucinations, in which he repeatedly heard his great-grandma talking to him. She felt alarmed by this possible psychotic feature. With some preparation and the supervisor's help, the therapist called Juan and told him that she now knew how she failed to understand him and asked Juan to give her another chance. In the following session, the therapist expressed her interest in knowing more about his communication with his great-grandma, among other things. Juan shared information about some rituals and practices of his Vodou religion and became excited when he felt the therapist believed him and saw his "hallucination" as common, normal, and honored in his religion. This rupture-repair process significantly deepened the emotional working bond between them.

Strengths- and Resource-Based Conceptualization and Interventions

From the general psychological literature, especially on motivation (e.g., Leary, 2007), self-efficacy (Maddux, 2005), and positive psychology (Boniwell, 2012), we can derive the understanding that the mechanism for change is rooted in positive self-perception, emotion, and energy, and so is the ability to trust and form relationships. This understanding has gradually been integrated into psychotherapy. The tradition of applying medical or disease models in psychotherapy has turned out to be more problematic than effective (Elkins, 2007) and even more problematic to racial/ethnic minority clients (Sue & Sue, 2015). Learning both wisdom and lessons from the psychological literature, it is therapeutically strategic to focus on enhancing client positive experiences and qualities in therapy. The strengths- and resource-based therapeutic approaches involve identifying and building clients' capacities for growth, problem-solving, adjustment, and the desire to be and do good (Conoley & Scheel, 2018). The aims of such practice include both the traditionally valued symptom reduction and well-being improvement. My clinical observation has convinced me of its potential in facilitating clients' sense of consensus and collaboration inherent in the working alliance and their motivation for and self-efficacy in pursuing desired changes in and out of therapy sessions. Just as Dr. Martin Luther King Jr. once said, "Darkness cannot drive out darkness; only light can do that." It is desirable that therapists help clients see more light during difficult times.

Therapists' recognition of client strength can be empowering, particularly for racial and ethnic minority clients who may have endured unwarranted oppression and negative perceptions and evaluations in life. Furthermore, focusing more on well-being than on pathology in conceptualization and more on building the working alliance and uncovering strength than on direct symptom removal may help prevent unintentional harm, which mostly occurs through inappropriate diagnosis and problematic interventions (Jarrett, 2008). The therapist–client bond is more likely when clients feel positive and capable of trusting. I believe that behind every symptom is the client's desire for positive change and effort to cope. It is the therapists' responsibility to help them discover and expand this positive energy and strength. In practice, one may consider using these reminders: (1) don't be overoccupied by client problems, but focus on seeing clients as holistic persons and view their presented problems as contextual information to facilitate an accurate understanding; (2) don't overfocus on the analysis of clients' problems (which makes the therapist, not the client, an expert) but on helping them discover their strengths and resources in the context of their problems; (3) don't overfocus on solving clients' problems (only clients can solve their problems) but on helping them gain motivation, freedom, and the ability to solve their problems; (4) don't overfocus on convincing clients that they are sick and educating them about their illness but on helping them see and utilize their positive desire, abilities, and personal qualities underneath their symptoms to move toward healing and health; and (5) don't overfocus on "going deeper" at the expense of the client's pain (which can lead to helpless feelings) but on helping them alleviate unwanted pain by recognizing contextual triggers as well as resources in their personal experience.

Summary

Effective psychotherapy for racial/ethnic minority clients depends on the quality and strength of the therapist–client working alliance. Hence it is essential and strategic that therapists be prepared for and focus on facilitating the therapeutic bond with clients and gaining client collaboration in therapeutic goals and tasks throughout the therapy process. To develop necessary competencies, therapist may need to engage in deliberative learning and practice. Considering the differential social and cultural realities for individuals of diverse racial/ethnic backgrounds in our society, therapists should feel motivated to understand both themselves and their clients in diverse social contexts, in which the system of privilege and oppression impacts people differently. Thus, a therapist deliberatively learning to connect with ethnic minority clients includes doing the needed self-work that allows him or her to develop appreciation for cultural diversity and cultivate respect for clients with different social realities. This work can be done in multiple ways, such as intentionally learning about the life and social experiences of ethnic minorities, overcoming prejudice and negative stereotypes toward them, and intentionally working to correct implicit biases about them. With appreciation and respect, therapists further develop the characteristics of being open-minded, accepting, honest, and empathic, and they facilitate developing the working alliance with racial/ethnic minority clients.

Deliberative practice of specific therapeutic skills can also be of great help to enhance a therapist's ability in strengthening the working alliance with ethnic minority clients. There are various ways in which such practice can be conducted. To provide some heuristic examples, this chapter discussed how deliberate and intentional effort may enhance the therapist's ability in understanding and taking diverse client perspectives, being culturally humble, and using strength-based conceptualizations and interventions. As shown by the clinical examples, therapeutic skills may be important vehicles in reaching ethnic minority clients, gaining their trust, and leading to the development of a healthy working alliance.

References

Ackerman, S. J., & Hilsenroth, M. J. (2001). A review of therapist characteristics and techniques negatively impacting the therapeutic alliance. *Psychotherapy: Theory, Research, Practice, Training, 38*, 171185.

Ackerman, S. J., & Hilsenroth, M. J. (2003). A review of therapist characteristics and techniques positively impacting the therapeutic alliance. *Clinical Psychological Review, 23*, 133.

Altman, N. (2007). Toward the acceptance of human similarity and difference. In J. C. Muran (Ed.), *Dialogues on difference: Studies of diversity in the therapeutic relationship* (pp. 15–25). Washington DC: APA Publisher.

American Psychological Association (2016). A new look at racial and ethnic disparities in mental health care. Retrieved from https://www.apa.org/monitor/2016/01/publication-disparities.aspx

Banaji, M. (2018). The mind is a difference-seeking machine: An interview with Krista Tippett. Retrieved from https://onbeing.org/programs/mahzarin-banaji-the-mind-is-a-difference-seeking-machine-aug2018/

Betancourt, H., & Lopez, S. R. (1993). The study of culture, ethnicity, and race in American psychology. *American Psychologist, 48,* 629–637.

Blair, I. V., Steiner, J. F., Fairclough, D. L., Hanratty, R., Price, D. W., Hirsh, H. K., . . . Havranek, E. P. (2013). Clinicians' implicit ethnic/racial bias and perceptions of care among Black and Latino patients. *Annals of Family Medicine, 11,* 43–52.

Blow, F. C., Zeber, J. E., McCarthy, J. F., Valenstein, M., Gillon, L., & Bingham, C. R. (2004). Ethnicity and diagnostic patterns in veterans with psychoses. *Social Psychiatry & Psychiatric Epidemiology, 39*(10), 841–851.

Boniwell, I. (2012). *Positive psychology in a nutshell: The science of happiness* (3rd ed.). London: McGraw-Hill.

Brondolo, E., Byer, K., Gianaros, P. J., Liu, C., Prather, A. A., Thomas, K., & Woods-Giscombé, C. L. (2017). Stress and health disparities: Contexts, mechanisms, and interventions among racial/ethnic minority and low socioeconomic status populations. American Psychological Association. Retrieved from https://www.apa.org/pi/health-disparities/resources/stress-report.pdf

Brown, L. M., Bradley, M. M., & Lang, P. J. (2006). Affective reactions to pictures of ingroup and outgroup members. *Biological Psychology, 71,* 303–311.

Brown, T. N., Williams, D. R., Jackson, J. S., Neighbors, H. W., Torres, M., Sellers, S. L., & Brown, K. T. (2000). "Being Black and feeling blue": The mental health consequences of racial discrimination. *Race and Society, 2,* 117–131.

Bussing, R., & Gary, F. A. (2012). Eliminating mental health disparities by 2020: Everyone's actions matter. *Journal of the American Academy of Child & Adolescent Psychiatry, 51*(7), 663–666. https://doi.org/10.1016/j.jaac.2012.04.005

Castonguay, L. G., Constantino, M. J., & Holtforth, M. G. (2006). The working alliance: Where are we and where should we go? *Psychotherapy: Theory, Research, Practice, Training, 43*(3), 271–279. http://dx.doi.org/10.1037/0033-3204.43.3.271

Castonguay, L. G., & Hill, C. E. (2017). *How and why are some therapists better than others?* Washington DC: American Psychological Association Press

Coates, T. (2015). *Between the world and me.* New York: Random House Spiegel & Grau.

Conoley, C., & Scheel, M. (2018). *Goal focused positive psychotherapy.* New York: Oxford University Press.

Crenshaw, K. W. (1989). Mapping the margins: Intersectionality, identity politics, and violence against women of color. An essay. Retrieved from https://www.racialequitytools.org/resourcefiles/mapping-margins.pdf

Duan, C., & Brown, C. (2015). *Becoming a multiculturally competent counselor.* Thousand Oaks, CA: Sage.

Duan, C., & Sager, K. (2018). Understanding empathy: Current state and future research challenges. In C. R. Snyder, S. J. Lopez, L. M. Edwards, & S. C. Marques (Eds.), *Oxford handbook of positive psychology, 3rd Ed.* New York: Oxford University Press. doi:10.1093/oxfordhb/9780199396511.013.62

Elkins, D. N. (2007). The medical model in psychotherapy: Its limitations and failures. *Journal of Humanistic Psychology, 49*(1), 66–84. https://doi.org/10.1177/0022167807307901

Fitzpatrick, M. R., Iwakabe, S., & Stalikas, A. (2005). Perspective divergence in the working alliance. *Psychotherapy Research, 15*(1–2), 69–80. https://doi.org/10.1080/10503300512331327056

Gager, F. P. (2004). Exploring relationships among termination status, therapy outcome and client satisfaction. *Dissertation Abstracts International: Section B: The Sciences and Engineering, 64* (7-B), 3522. (Abstract number 2004-99002-141)

Godfrey, E. B., Santos, C. E., & Burson, E. (2017). For better or worse? System-justifying beliefs in sixth-grade predict trajectories of self-esteem and behavior across early adolescence. *Child Development*. Retrieved from https://doi-org.www2.lib.ku.edu/10.1111/cdev.12854

Goldman, H. H. (2012). Taking issue. *Psychiatric Services, 63,* 847.

Gonzalez, C. M., Deno, M. L., Kintzer, E., Marantz, P. R., Lypson, M. L., & McKee, M. D. (2018). Patient perspectives on racial and ethnic implicit bias in clinical encounters: Implications for curriculum development. *Patient Education and Counseling, 101,* 1669–1675. https://doi.org/10.1016/j.pec.2018.05.016

Goodman, D. J. (2015). Oppression and privilege: Two sides of the same coin. *Journal of Intercultural Communication, 18,* 1–14.

Greenberg, L. S. (1986). Change process research. *Journal of Constructivist Psychology, 54*(1), 4–9. https://doi.org/10.1080/10503307.2014.906764

Hatcher, R., & Barends, A. W. (2006). How a return to theory could help alliance research. *Psychotherapy, 43,* 292–299. doi:10.1037/0033-3204.43.3.292

Hays, P. (2016). *Addressing cultural complexities in practice* (3rd ed.). Washington DC: American Psychological Association Press.

Heinonen, E. (2014). Therapists' professional and personal characteristics as predictors of working alliance and outcome in psychotherapy. Helsinki, Finland: National Institute for Health and Welfare. Retrieved from https://www.julkari.fi/bitstream/handle/10024/114948/URN_ISBN_978-952-302-127-3.pdf?sequence=1

Hersoug, A. G., Monsen, J. T., Havik, O. E., & Hoglend, P. (2000, June). Prediction of early working alliance: Diagnoses, relationship, and interpsychic variables as predictors. Paper presented at the Society for Psychotherapy Research, Chicago.

Holbrook, C., Fessler, D. M. T., & Navarrete, C. (2016). Looming large in others' eyes: Racial stereotypes illuminate dual adaptations for representing threat versus prestige as physical size. *Evolution & Human Behavior, 37,* 67–78.

Hook, J. N., Davis, D. E., Owen, J., Worthington, E. L., Jr., & Utsey, S. O. (2013). Cultural humility: Measuring openness to culturally diverse clients. *Journal of Counseling Psychology, 60,* 353–366. doi:10.1037/a0032595

Horvath, A. O., & Bedi, R. P. (2002). The alliance. In J. C. Norcross (Ed.), *Psychotherapy relationships that work. Therapist contributions and responsiveness to clients* (pp. 37–70). New York: Oxford University Press

Jacobson, A. (2015). Examples of implicit racial bias at work. Feminist philosophers. Retrieved from https://feministphilosophers.wordpress.com/2015/01/04/examples-of-implicit-racial-bias-at-work/

Jarrett, C. (2008). When therapy causes harm. The Psychologist . . . The British Psychological Society: Promoting excellence in psychology. Retrieved from https://thepsychologist.bps.org.uk/volume-21/edition-1/when-therapy-causes-harm

Kraus, D. R., Castonguay, L. G., Boswell, J. F., Nordberg, S. S., & Hayes, J. A. (2011). Therapist effectiveness: Implications for accountability and patient care. *Psychotherapy Research, 21,* 267–276.

Leary M. R. (2007). Motivation and emotional aspects of the self. *Annual Review of Psychology, 58*, 317–44.

Lichenberg, J. W., Wettersten, K. B., Mull, H., Moberly, R. L., Merkey, K. B., & Corey, A. T. (1988). Relationship and control as correlates of psychotherapy quality and outcome. *Journal of Consulting and Clinical Psychology, 45*, 322–337.

Martin, D. J., Garske, J. P., & Davis, M. K. (2000). Relation of the therapeutic alliance with outcome and other variables: A meta-analytic review. *Journal of Consulting and Clinical Psychology, 68*(3), 438–450. http://dx.doi.org/10.1037/0022-006X.68.3.438

Maddux, J. E. (2005). Self-efficacy: The power of believing you can. In C.R Snyder & S. J. Lopez (Eds.), *Handbook of positive psychology* (pp. 227–287). New York: Oxford University Press.

McGuire, T. G., & Miranda, J. (2008). New evidence regarding racial and ethnic disparities in mental health: Policy implications. *Health Affairs, 27*(2), 393–403. https://doi.org/10.1377/hlthaff.27.2.393

Nissen-Lie, H. A., Monsen, T., & Ronnestad, M. H. (2010). Therapist predictors of early patient-rated working alliance: A multilevel approach. *Psychotherapy Research, 20*, 627–646. doi:10.1080/10503307.2010.497633

Owen, J., Tao, K. W., Drinane, J. M., Hook, J., Davis, D., & Kune, N. F. (2016). Client perceptions of therapists' multicultural orientation: Cultural (missed) opportunities and cultural humility. *Professional Psychology: Research and Practice, 47*(1), 30–37. doi:10.1037/pro0000046

Page, D., & Shepherd, H. (2010). The sociology of discrimination: Racial discrimination in employment, housing, credit, and consumer. *Annual Review of Sociology, 34*, 181–209.

Ramanathan, C. S. (2014, January). What does globalization got to do with cultural competence, social development, and ethics? Plenary speech presented at the International Conference on Bounds of Ethics, Christ University, Bangalore, India.

Rogers, C. (1980). *A way of being*. Boston: Houghton Mifflin.

Rogers, C. (1986). Carl Rogers on the development of the person-centered approach. *Person-Centered Review, 1*(3), 257–259.

Satcher, D. (2001). Preface. Mental health: Culture, race, and ethnicity: A supplement to Mental Health: A Report of the Surgeon General. Retrieved from https://www.ncbi.nlm.nih.gov/books/NBK44248/

Schwartz, R. C., & Blankenship, D. M. (2014). Racial disparities in psychotic disorder diagnosis: A review of empirical literature. *World Journal of Psychiatry, 4*(4), 133–140.

Sexton, H. (1996). Process, life events, and symptomatic change in brief eclectic psychotherapy. *Journal of Consulting and Clinical Psychology, 64*, 1358–1365

Smedley, B. D., Stith, A. Y., & Nelson, A. R. (Eds.). (2003). *Unequal treatment: Confronting racial and ethnic disparities in health care*. Washington, DC: National Academies Press.

Smith, T. B., & Trimble, J. E. (2016). Culturally adapted mental health services: An updated meta-analysis of client outcomes. In J. E. Trimble & T. B. Smith (Eds.), *Foundations of multicultural psychology: Research to inform effective practice* (pp. 129–144). Washington, DC: American Psychological Association.

Stiles, W. B. (2002). Session Evaluation Questionnaire: Structure and use. Retrieved from http://www.users.muohio.edu/stileswb/session_evaluation_questionnaire.html

Strupp, H. H. (1998). The Vanderbilt I Study revisited. *Psychotherapy Research, 8*, 17–29. doi:10.1093/ptr/8.1.17

Sue, D. W. (2003). Cultural competence in the treatment of ethnic minority populations. In Council of National Psychological Associations for the Advancement of Ethnic Minority Interests (Ed.), *Psychological treatment of ethnic minority populations* (pp. 4–7). Washington DC: Association of Black Psychologists. Retrieved from http://www.apa.org/pi/oema/resources/brochures/treatment-minority.pdf

Sue, D. W., & Sue, D. (2015). Counseling the culturally diverse. Hoboken, NJ: Wiley.

Tervalon, M., & Murray-Garcia, J. (1998). Cultural humility versus cultural competence: A critical distinction in defining physician training outcomes in multicultural education. *Journal of Health Care for the Poor and Underserved, 9*(2), 117–125.

Tropp, L. R., & Godsil, R. D. (2015). Overcoming implicit bias and racial anxiety. Retrieved from https://www.psychologytoday.com/us/blog/sound-science-sound-policy/201501/overcoming-implicit-bias-and-racial-anxiety

Wampold, B. E., & Brown, G. S. (2005). Estimating variability in outcomes attributable to therapists: A naturalistic study of outcomes in managed care. *Journal of Consulting and Clinical Psychology, 73*(5), 914–923.

8

A Therapist's Guide to Repairing Ruptures in the Working Alliance

Jerald R. Gardner, Lauren M. Lipner, Catherine F. Eubanks,
and J. Christopher Muran

In this chapter, we present a skill set aimed at helping beginning and advanced therapists to recognize and identify therapeutic misattunements (termed "ruptures" in the empirical literature; Safran, Muran, & Samstag, 1994), and we present a framework for managing these difficult moments in psychotherapy. Our overall aim is to provide a set of tools for therapists to use in real-world clinical problems as they develop a working alliance with their clients. And, last, we encourage the reader to take a deep breath! These rupture moments are common in psychotherapy, and we hope to instill a sense of optimism and competence when you encounter them in your clinical travels.

The Working Alliance

Interpersonal problems in psychotherapy have long been the subject of study and discussion. Sigmund Freud's early conception of his patients' negative reactions toward him were identified as "resistance" (Freud, 1927). Subsequent clinical theorists created other terms to describe their experiences of difficult moments in psychotherapy, such as "enactments" (Jacobs, 1986), "misattunements" (The Boston Change Process Study Group, 2010), "empathic failures" (Kohut, 1984), and "impasses," (Hill, Nutt-Williams, Heaton, Thompson, & Rhodes, 1996), to name a few.

With psychotherapy increasing in prominence in the twentieth century, leaders in the field began to identify language to describe the psychotherapy process as it relates to both the therapist *and* the client, and not solely the client. The concept of the "therapeutic alliance" was first introduced by Lester Luborsky in 1976, who defined it as the client's view of the therapist as a supportive figure, as well as a shared sense of joint responsibility in working to achieve the client's goals (Luborsky, 1976). Edward Bordin reformulated the concept of the alliance in 1979 and termed it the "working alliance." Bordin's goal—with his reformulated alliance concept—was to explore mechanisms of clinical change that could account for different theoretical orientations (i.e., psychoanalytic psychotherapy, behaviorism, etc.) (Bordin, 1979).

Bordin speculated that strong alliances in therapy resulted from the negotiations of expectations between the therapist and client. He saw these negotiations as occurring on two fronts: the therapist's clinical expectations of the client and the client's understanding of his or her own problems. He further identified three components to this negotiation: (1) the therapist's and client's agreement on the goals of what should be the focus of the therapy, (2) their collaboration on tasks to achieve those goals, and (3) the establishment of an affective "bond" between the two (Bordin, 1979). This definition paved the way for the development of research assessments that could track the client's subjective experience of the working alliance, such as the widely used Working Alliance Inventory (Horvath & Greenberg, 1989).

Bordin viewed the alliance construct as the movement toward a purposeful collaboration between therapist and client. Clinically, Bordin's conceptualization of the alliance can serve as an anchor for both the client's and therapist's moment-to-moment experiences in the therapy. Questions such as "Are we collaborating together on a shared goal?," "Does the therapy feel like we are working together toward a common purpose, or does it feel like we have conflicting ideas of the therapy?," and "How do I feel about my client?" illustrate the usefulness of Bordin's alliance definition as it pertains to clinical use. These questions, while not necessarily explicitly shared with the client, are useful as a therapist's "gauge" in determining the overall health of the working alliance and whether or not an alliance rupture (see later discussion for more on this topic) (Safran et al., 1994), a misattunement, or a misunderstanding in therapeutic process has occurred. Presently, the working alliance (agreement on goals, agreement on tasks, and the affective bond in the dyad) has long been linked to treatment outcome in a host of studies and meta-analytic reviews (Flückiger, Del Re, Wampold, Symonds, & Horvath, 2012; Horvath & Symonds, 1991; Horvath, Del Re, Flückiger, & Symonds, 2011; Martin et al., 2000).

Therapeutic Ruptures: Definition and Historical Perspectives

In the late 1980s, Jeremy Safran launched a research program on the working alliance. As the working alliance came to be better understood as a significant aspect for clients' successes or failures in therapy, the program focused on understanding "ruptures"—simply defined as "an impairment or fluctuation in the quality of the alliance between the therapist and client" (Safran, Crocker,

McMain, & Murray, 1990, p. 154). Early research in defining the concept of a rupture identified several interpersonal processes indicative of problems in the working alliance. Notably, Safran, Muran, and colleagues identified a marker to highlight a rupture, defined as the therapist and client engaging in some kind of a negative process (see Safran et al., 1994).

But what did these "negative processes" actually look like? How would one know that a rupture was occurring, and how would a therapist know when they had stepped into a rupture? Refinements to their early work began to identify specific therapeutic events that were indicative of rupture occurrence. Specifically, Safran, Muran, and colleagues began to focus on two categories of events indicative of a rupture developing. These were termed *withdrawal ruptures* and *confrontation ruptures* (Safran & Muran, 1996; Safran & Muran, 2000; Harper, 1989a, 1989b). Withdrawal ruptures encapsulated a negative therapeutic movement *away* from the other, while confrontation ruptures involved a negative therapeutic movement *against* the other. A breakdown of these two different types of rupture types is illustrated in Table 8.1.

Safran and Muran began to develop the structure of these rupture categories. Withdrawal markers were noted to be subtle movements *away* from the therapist and as potentially easily overlooked. By contrast, confrontation ruptures involved client movements *against* the therapist and could be thought of as efforts of control or aggression (Safran & Muran, 2000). Safran and Muran further identified conditions that may influence whether a client engages in a withdrawal

Table 8.1 Rupture types as expressed by the client

Withdrawal ruptures	Confrontation ruptures
Sudden silence in the therapy	Complaints about personal qualities of the therapist
Minimal responses from the client	Complaints about the therapist's competency
Sudden topic shifts in the therapeutic content	Disagreement about the activities (or tasks) of the therapy
Abstract or intellectualized speech from the client	Questioning of the client's own participation in therapy
Storytelling or tangential references that detract from the therapy	Disagreement over the parameters of the therapy
Overly protective or accommodating behaviors from the client	Complaints about the client's overall progress in therapy
Begrudging acceptance on the part of the client	

versus a confrontation rupture. The two rupture categories reflect clients' dia-lectical needs in relationships, namely, the client's need to feel related to others that can be achieved by "withdrawal" into the self (avoidance) or away from self (appeasement), and the need for self-definition or agency that can be achieved through confronting the other (by attacks or control). For example, a client may suddenly become silent in the treatment or begrudgingly go along with the ther-apist (withdrawal rupture), which may mark an avoidance of expression of his or her true feelings (in this example, the client's true feelings may be that the therapy is not actually helpful), which serves to maintain the client's relatedness to the therapist. Conversely, a client may suddenly voice a disagreement about the activities or the tasks of the therapy, an example being when a client voices her thoughts on the uselessness of a thought record exercise (confrontation rupture). This move may be seen as a movement by the client to assert her own agency in relation to the therapist (Safran & Muran, 2000). Taken together, with-drawal and confrontation ruptures represent interpersonal processes occurring between client and therapist, and they reflect moment-to-moment experiences in psychotherapy (i.e., a therapist may make a statement that inadvertently makes the client feel misunderstood, and the client subsequently becomes silent and withdraws as a result).

In a similar vein, ruptures may be expressed by *therapists* in similar and sometimes complementary ways. Therapists may find themselves withdrawing from the therapeutic work with their mind wandering, or they may suddenly shift the topic of the therapy (withdrawal ruptures). They may also find them-selves putting down their clients or insulting them, in overt and sometimes co-vert ways or by inadvertently forcing their client to conform to their expectations of the therapy or their theoretical understanding of their issues (confrontation ruptures) (Muran & Eubanks, in press). For the purposes of this chapter, we will focus on ruptures that are expressed by the client.

Contemporary research in the usefulness of identifying ruptures in psycho-therapy has found that the therapist's ability to recognize and attend to these rupture moments has a significant relationship to client improvement at the end of therapy in a host of measurable domains (depression symptoms, personality disorder symptoms, resolution of presenting complaints for therapy, and social adjustment, to name a few) (Safran, Muran, & Eubanks-Carter, 2011). Stiles and colleagues similarly found that a therapist's attentiveness to ruptures in treatment and the ability to engage with clients during these difficult moments was associ-ated with more significant clinical gains once therapy ended (Stiles et al. 2004). Most recently, a meta-analysis by Eubanks and colleagues found that ruptures that were successfully attended to by therapists resulted in a significant relation-ship, with both symptom reduction at the end of treatment and an increased likelihood that the client completed treatment and did not drop out (Eubanks,

Muran, & Safran, 2018). Over time, as the significance of ruptures became apparent in their impact on psychotherapy, this strategy of the therapist's attempts to address the rupture with his or her client and restore the working alliance was termed *rupture repair* and became a significant focus of research (Safran, Muran, Samstag, & Stevens, 2002).

An illuminating recent review of rupture repair strategies surveyed peer-nominated experts in psychotherapy (psychologists and social workers of various theoretical orientations) and identified effective rupture repair strategies. Overall, strategies they considered effective included the therapist's exploration of the client's experience of the rupture and the therapist's acknowledgment of the client's perspective (Eubanks, Burckell, & Goldfried, 2018).

Interest in defining how therapists could repair ruptures in therapy has subsequently garnered considerable interest in the field. Bennett, Parry, and Ryle (2006) found that, in more successful therapy cases, therapists were better able to recognize a rupture, while in less successful therapy outcomes, therapists were less able to notice a rupture in the alliance. Several studies have also noted the impact of "alliance-focused supervision" on helping novice therapists navigate ruptures. This training involved helping therapists develop a greater awareness of interpersonal dynamics impacting the working alliance (Bambling, King, Raue, Schweittzer, & Lambert, 2006) and helping therapists to encourage their clients to express their feelings about interpersonal problems (Crits-Christoph et al., 2006; Muran, Samstag, Safran, & Winston, 2005).

Levendosky and colleagues additionally found that observer-rated in-session behaviors between therapist and client were helpful in improving therapists' abilities to navigate ruptures (Levendosky & Hopwood, 2017). Similarly, Lambert found that ongoing assessments of the client's self-reported symptom severity, with feedback delivered to the therapist, resulted in an improved ability on the part of the therapist to recognize that the treatment was heading in a negative direction, thereby providing an opportunity for the therapist to "turn the treatment course around" (Lambert, 2015). Last, Anderson and colleagues found that therapists' "facilitative interpersonal skills" (i.e., emotional expression, hopefulness, and empathy, to name a few) were related to greater symptom reduction in their clients than therapists who rated low on facilitative interpersonal skills (Anderson, McClintock, Himawan, Song, & Patterson, 2016). The multitude of different research approaches began to highlight the interest in understanding the phenomenology of ruptures and their subsequent repairs because these were perceived to have a direct relationship with improvements in psychotherapy.

In the next section, we focus in on our model, which is known as the *rupture repair model* (see Figure 8.1) (Safran & Muran, 2000; Muran, Safran, & Eubanks-Carter, 2010). This model is the culmination of substantial research toward a better understanding of the process of ruptures in therapy and their successful

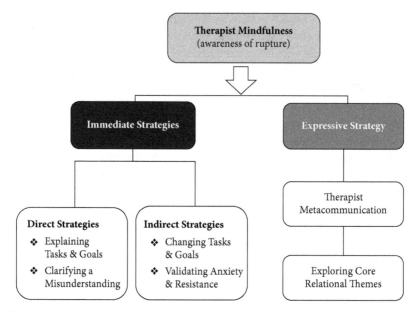

Figure 8.1 Rupture repair model.

repairs. It is also the current and revised version of our early model known as the "stage-process model," which identified markers of a rupture event taking place (Safran, et al., 1994). The rupture repair model has demonstrated effectiveness in greater therapist expressiveness in-session and lower levels of client avoidance in therapy, and these have been linked to improved overall alliance (Muran, Safran, Eubanks, & Gorman, 2018). It has also been linked to reduced dropout rates among clients (Muran et al., 2005) and an increase in friendly and welcoming behaviors from therapists, the latter being important in facilitating clients' self-assertion and abilities to discuss and bring up ruptures in therapy (Safran et al., 2014). The development of our model was empirically driven and was influenced by research from other groups, one of which experimented with changing in-session tasks as a method to address ruptures (Aspland, Llewelyn, Hardy, Barkham, & Stiles, 2008). Our overarching goal in developing the model is to help therapists recognize ruptures as they occur in real time in-session and then to pivot to using a set of intervention skills to attempt a repair of the rupture.

A word on the phenomenology of ruptures: the rupture repair model is founded on the premise that ruptures occur naturally in therapy and that such occurrences are inevitable. This premise was influenced by several theorists who note the importance of understanding the "other" in therapy (Aron, 1996;

Benjamin, 1990). From this vantage point, ruptures are not seen as interpersonal experiences to be avoided altogether but rather as experiences that, when successfully navigated, can bring about a feeling of mutual recognition and healing in the therapy.

Mindfulness

A gateway and first step to recognizing ruptures in our rupture repair model (Figure 8.1) is through the therapeutic technique of *mindfulness* (Safran & Muran, 2000). We encourage therapists to practice mindfulness outside of therapy, particularly in clinical supervision if they have access to a supervisor trained in mindfulness-based therapeutic techniques. If the therapist does not have access to a supervisor trained in mindfulness, additional information about the use of mindfulness in psychotherapy can be found at https://www.apa.org/monitor/2012/07-08/ce-corner.aspx.

Development of the mindfulness skill serves several functions: it deepens the therapist's awareness of their own internal reactions to their clients, thereby making it easier for the therapist to recognize ruptures that occur in the therapy, and, by extension, practicing mindfulness promotes an awareness of the internal reactions of the client. As ruptures in therapy can often take the form of subtle interactions, mindfulness is particularly useful in this regard. It should be viewed as a tool to help therapists *recognize* that a rupture has taken place or may be in the process of occurring. Our stance is that mindfulness can be thought of as a pan-theoretical, technical strategy that can work in concert with different schools of psychotherapy.

Mindfulness is a simple though immensely important exercise in sharpening therapists' awareness of their own moment-to-moment internal thinking and emotional states, and it can also help with the therapist's practice of tolerating negative emotions. There are variations on mindfulness scripts, though our mindfulness practice involves three main components: (1) direction of attention, (2) remembering, and (3) nonjudgmental awareness (Safran & Muran, 2000). *Direction of attention* refers to an awareness of when one's mind begins to wander and the active process of returning attention to a focal point. *Remembering* refers to the act of remembering that, as the therapist, your attention has moved to another aspect of the therapy without your conscious awareness. *Nonjudgmental awareness* refers to the ability to observe the contents of one's mind without pushing uncomfortable or unrelated thoughts or feeling states out of awareness; the overall goal being for the therapist to return to a mindful frame of mind without becoming lost in self-judgment (Safran & Muran, 2000).

The following is a typical mindfulness script used in our own group supervision sessions aimed at enhancing trainee therapists' mindfulness skills.

Mindfulness Skill-Building Demonstration

This session takes approximately 5 minutes to complete.

SUPERVISOR: Let's start by getting into a comfortable position, uncross your legs, and place your feet on the floor. Rest your hands on your lap. Close your eyes.

SUPERVISOR: Go ahead and take three, even breaths.

SUPERVISOR: And now just go ahead and breathe normally; let your breathing find its own natural rhythm. While you're breathing, focus your attention on your breath.

SUPERVISOR: Trace with your mind the flow of air as you breathe in and then back out again. Notice how the process of breathing feels, and notice the physical sensations as you breathe in and back out again.

SUPERVISOR: If you notice any sounds in this room, or outside of this room, simply acknowledge their presence, and then bring your attention back to your breath.

SUPERVISOR: Imagine for a moment that you're sitting in a movie theater in front of a large movie screen. If thoughts or feelings enter your mind, whether positive or negative, imagine that you can see them on the screen in front of you. Notice what they look like, what form they take. Go ahead and let the images on the screen pass, and let them go.

SUPERVISOR: Every once in a while, gently return your attention to your breathing.

SUPERVISOR: Now go ahead and take three even breaths.

SUPERVISOR: When you're ready, you can open your eyes and come back to the room.

With the practice of mindfulness in supervision and outside of psychotherapy, the goal for the trainee is to become more aware of their own internal affective states and thought processes, a skill that can subsequently be generalized to their experiences in psychotherapy. The ultimate goal is for the trainee therapist to begin to be more mindful in-session to their own affective states, feelings toward their clients, moments of dissociation where their own mind begins to "wander," feelings of boredom with their client, and so on.

Next is a hypothetical example of a therapist using mindfulness skills in-session during a difficult client encounter.

Mindfulness Example In-Session

THERAPIST: How are you doing this week?

CLIENT: I'm doing okay, I went to visit my mom at her apartment and she's doing fine.

THERAPIST: How is she holding up?

CLIENT: She's all right, you know, nothing new to report.

THERAPIST: And how are you?

CLIENT: I'm okay, just going through the motions.

[Through mindfulness and observing her own reactions, the therapist begins to notice that she is uncomfortable with the client's minimal responses at the outset of therapy.]

THERAPIST: I wanted to check in on your depression symptoms; how's your mood been lately? Has it been hard to get up in the morning and get moving?

CLIENT: I've been doing all right. I guess I've been feeling a little better, and I've been able to get up easier in the morning.

THERAPIST: That's good. I think if you're able to make some small movements to start your day, it will get a little easier to tackle the next task, and you'll find your energy levels starting to return.

[Therapist becomes aware of talking in an "expert" way, something she doesn't usually do with this client.]

CLIENT: Okay, good to know.

THERAPIST: You know, I just realized that I'm doing a lot of talking in this session, and usually that doesn't happen. I'm wondering if you noticed that, too?

CLIENT: Not sure what you mean?

THERAPIST: Maybe I'm filling a lot more of the space in here today because you seem to be more quiet.

CLIENT: Yeah, it's been a hard week for me. I guess I don't really want to talk about it.

THERAPIST: Okay, I understand. Maybe it's more important for us to sit with the fact that it's been a hard week for you.

In this example, through the therapist's own use of mindfulness, she becomes aware of two things: (1) she begins to feel discomfort when her client from the outset of therapy is minimally engaging and speaking, and (2) she begins to be aware of talking in an "expert" voice when she starts to talk about depression symptoms and the client's energy level. She simultaneously becomes aware that this is an unusual occurrence for her with this client and that she doesn't normally take on this "professional" role with the client. As a result of this awareness, the therapist recognizes that her client has withdrawn from her in this session (withdrawal rupture) and that this occurrence may be indicative of a rupture. The therapist's awareness of the withdrawal rupture is a skill that has been developed through the contributing factor of the therapist's own mindfulness practice and her attunement to her own internal states as she interacts with her client. This attunement is an important component in the therapist's recognizing that a rupture has just occurred, and continual mindfulness practice works to enhance this attunement in the therapy.

The therapist then shifts to the exploration of her client's withdrawal behaviors and her resulting behaviors. As demonstrated in the preceding example, mindfulness acts as a type of therapeutic "radar," so to speak, that can be used by a therapist to scan their own personal and internal reactions to their clients and their own emotions as they relate to ruptures that occur in therapy.

Immediate Strategies (Direct)

Once the therapist has become mindful of the fact that a rupture has occurred, the rupture repair model identifies the decision point of choosing either an *immediate* or *expressive* intervention strategy to address the rupture based on the characteristics of the rupture that has just occurred. In general, immediate strategies promote an immediate intervention to address the rupture at hand; conversely, the expressive strategy promotes a depth-oriented process of expression of the client's needs and a discussion of the therapist's own contributions to the rupture. For example, if a client expresses confusion about the tasks and the goals of the therapy, the therapist may opt to try an *immediate* intervention strategy of explaining the tasks and goals. By contrast, a rupture may call for a more in-depth strategy to explore larger interpersonal processes between the therapist and client and may be more beneficial to the client's progress in therapy depending on the clinical context. These strategies will be contrasted in further detail in later examples.

Direct rupture repair interventions involve the therapist's attempt to directly address the rupture with the client. In the rupture repair model, this type of intervention may take the form of (1) explaining the tasks and goals of the therapy or (2) clarifying a misunderstanding. An explanation of the tasks and goals of therapy addresses the rupture directly by reorienting the therapist and client to the goals of the therapy and/or the tasks intrinsic in reaching those goals.

Example of Explanation of Tasks and Goals (Direct Repair Strategy)

CLIENT: I didn't do the thought record from last week.

THERAPIST: Okay, that's fine. I'm curious if we could talk a bit to determine what happened and why you didn't do it.

CLIENT: Well, I just don't really know how helpful it is going to be to me.

THERAPIST: Can you say a little more about that?

CLIENT: Well, I guess I'm not sure what it's really supposed to be doing. I don't know how it's supposed to help me. [Rupture Statement: Disagreement about the activities (or tasks) of the therapy]

THERAPIST: Okay. Well, the basis of the thought record is to help to identify what you're thinking, what triggers those thoughts, and how those thoughts are ultimately connected to behaviors and feelings. [Direct Repair Strategy: Explanation of tasks and goals]
  When we spoke last week, you said that you were having difficulty separating out your thoughts and feelings. Was that the case?

CLIENT: Yeah, I think that's right, sometimes I find myself just overwhelmed with feelings and I break down.

THERAPIST: That sounds really frustrating. Let's try another thought record, and we can talk about what you're thinking and how those thoughts are connected to what you're feeling. I think it'll help us to get a better sense of your thought patterns and how those are connected to your emotions. [Direct Repair Strategy: Explanation of tasks and goals]

CLIENT: Okay, I'll give it another try.

In this example, the therapist does not move to change any of the tasks or goals of the therapy but instead works to explain the preexisting tasks and goals as they pertain to the therapeutic work. Explaining the tasks and goals of therapy is usually appropriate when there is genuine confusion from the client about how therapeutic activities work ultimately toward the client's goal. This strategy may be less effective in instances where a disagreement between therapist and client has occurred or hostility or tension is expressed by the client or the therapist. In those cases, a clarification or other intervention strategy may be more effective. An example of the intervention of clarifying a misunderstanding is presented next.

Example of Clarifying a Misunderstanding (Direct Repair Strategy)

CLIENT: I'm not really sure why I'm coming here, or what I'm getting out of this. [Rupture Statement: Questioning of the client's own participation in therapy]

THERAPIST: Can you say more about that? I want to make sure that I understand you.

CLIENT: Well, I've been coming here for about 2 months, and I thought I would start feeling less depressed, but I'm still feeling about the same. I'm not sure what we're working on.

THERAPIST: Hmm, okay. I hear that you've been feeling like this hasn't been helping you. I can imagine that's frustrating! But I'm glad you brought it up so that we can work on it. I'm a little confused, though, because it seemed to me like what we have been doing in here was helping you, is that right? I'm not sure and want to ask you, but that was my impression. We've been working on some behavioral activation tasks to help you feel more energized and motivated and to hopefully bring more pleasant emotions back into your life.

CLIENT: Well, it kind of helps me, for a little bit. But I'm still struggling with really negative thinking for a lot of my day. The activities help, but I'm still dealing with a lot of depression during the day. I guess maybe I had a hard time admitting that in here.

THERAPIST: Okay, so I think maybe we've missed something here. I thought the activities were a good place to start to help you feel more positive emotions and to help you get out of the house, but I'm hearing you say that that isn't enough and that you need more help. [Direct Repair Strategy: Clarifying a misunderstanding]

CLIENT: Yeah, that's about it.

THERAPIST: Maybe we can spend today's session talking about the negative thoughts that you're dealing with, and we can talk about some ways to manage those thoughts. [Direct Repair Strategy: Clarifying a misunderstanding]

CLIENT: Okay, I think that would be helpful.

The therapist believed that the behavioral activation exercises were addressing the client's depression symptoms to a satisfactory degree. By clarifying the misunderstanding, the therapist becomes aware of the fact that there is a misattunement in the room, and the therapist can work to correct the misunderstanding.

Immediate Strategies (Indirect)

Indirect rupture repair strategies differ from direct strategies in that they take a more subtle approach in addressing the rupture. Indirect strategies may be more useful during confrontation ruptures or when clients are affectively agitated or irritated. The indirect strategy of changing the tasks and/or goals addresses problems in the alliance and works to realign the client and therapist to get back on the same page with regard to the therapeutic work and its overall purpose.

Example of Changing the Tasks and Goals (Indirect Repair Strategy)

CLIENT: I was hanging out with some friends of mine over the weekend, and I started to wonder whether they really liked spending time with me. The more I thought about it, the more I couldn't get it out of my head, and I kept spinning all of these scenarios about wondering whether all of my relationships are like this, and whether anyone could really like me. . . . [Client begins to cry]

THERAPIST: I can see you're really upset. [Client continues to cry] Can you tell me what's happening for you right now?

CLIENT: I just . . . what you're saying makes sense to me in here, but I don't really know what I'm supposed to do with this information. [Rupture Statement: Disagreement about the activities (or tasks) of the therapy]

THERAPIST: I can tell that you're pretty upset right now, and part of me wants to explore what's making you so upset, but another part of me is hesitant to do that because it looks like you're in a lot of pain.

CLIENT: Yeah, I think I just continue to feel overwhelmed by these thoughts, and I understand more about where they're coming from and how they're connected to my past, but I don't really know how to stop them or how to just be normal.

THERAPIST: By "be normal," do you mean having less of these upsetting thoughts?

CLIENT: Yeah.

THERAPIST: I was thinking about something we said last week, about trying some mindfulness exercises in here. I think this could help you by practicing observing your thoughts and feelings from more of a nonjudgmental stance. [Indirect Repair Strategy: Therapist changes the task] With practice, you can become more skilled at detaching from your immediate experience without become lost in your thoughts. It may take a few weeks

of exercises in here for you to get the hang of it. What do you think? Want
to give it a shot?

CLIENT: Yeah, that makes sense. I'll give it a shot.

The crux of this intervention is to provide a course correction to change the
therapeutic tasks and/or goals and adjust the treatment in order to strengthen
the alliance. Ideally, the process of agreeing on new tasks and goals in the therapy
is a collaborative process in which both therapist and client participate. The collaboration on new tasks and goals then becomes a shared problem with a shared
solution.

The final indirect repair strategy consists of validating the client's anxiety and
resistance; it is particularly useful in de-escalating a negative interpersonal process between therapist and client and can be effective in addressing a confrontation rupture in which hostility is present. That said, it is equally as effective in
managing more subtle ruptures and withdrawal presentations. This is demonstrated in the following example.

Example of Validating the Client's Anxiety and Resistance (Indirect Repair Strategy)

CLIENT: I already told this to you last week! Don't you remember?

THERAPIST: I'm not sure I remember. . . .

CLIENT: I told you about my ex-husband's lying! I told you about how that
affected me! [Rupture Statement: Complaints about the therapist's
competency]

THERAPIST: I just want to take a step back here for a moment because I can tell
how angry you are at me, and I wonder if I've disappointed you in some
way. [Client remains silent] I have to say that I'd like to speak with you
more about this, but I'm a little hesitant to say anything because I can see
that I've really upset you. [Silence, client looks despondent] You look like
you want to say something.

CLIENT: I don't know, I'm just . . . tired of feeling this way.

THERAPIST: What way?

CLIENT: Just . . . lashing out at everyone. I just did it to you. It's happening eve-
rywhere. My eldest son won't even talk to me anymore.

THERAPIST: It's okay, it's all right for you to be angry in here. [Indirect Repair
Strategy: Therapist validates client's experience/anxiety]

The word "anxiety," as used in the intervention title, does not refer to symptoms of anxiety, per se, but rather to the client's anxious response that takes the form of confrontation. The therapeutic movement is to validate the client's emotional response and to recognize the distress that the client is experiencing, which creates a form of mutual recognition in the other and an experience of the client feeling seen and understood by the therapist.

Expressive Strategy (Exploring Core Relational Themes)

Taken together, these immediate rupture repair strategies, both direct and indirect, provide different maneuvers and options for managing ruptures with an immediate intervention. The rupture repair process can also follow what is known as an "expressive" intervention, in which the therapist attempts to explore core relational themes in the therapy. Certain clinical situations may call for an expressive rupture repair intervention. This type of intervention explores the therapist's own role in the rupture as well as the client's relational themes that may have been exacerbated or brought to the surface of the treatment through the rupture. This strategy is a broader attempt to examine relational functioning between therapist and client, and the therapist's use of the expressive strategy should take this into account.

Meta-Communication

After the therapist has become aware of the presence of a rupture, the expressive strategy first calls for the exploration of the rupture through the principle of *meta-communication*. The term is borrowed from Donald Kiesler (1996) and is defined as a communication about the communication process. Put another way, meta-communication is the therapist's ability to comment in real time about their own experience, thus sharing that experience with the client. Meta-communication is facilitated by the therapist's awareness of his or her own emotional states and internal experiences, a skill that is sharpened considerably during the therapist's own mindfulness experiences and exercises. It can be thought of as the therapist's translation of an aspect of the therapy they have become aware of in a clinically meaningful message to the client. A clinical example of meta-communication is highlighted in the following in-session example.

Expressive Strategy Stages

The structure of the expressive repair intervention (Safran & Muran, 2000) involves (1) the therapist recognizes that a rupture has occurred, (2) the therapist and client explore the rupture, and (3) the client expresses a need to the therapist. The imperative piece of this repair process is the second stage, in which the therapist attempts to understand the rupture process that has just occurred from a nondefensive and nonjudgmental stance. This can be a difficult process for the therapist as the client may be displaying anger, hostility, anxiety, disappointment, indifference, or any other host of powerful emotions toward the therapist. The therapeutic stance calls for the therapist to explore his or her contributions to the rupture while continuing to work to understand the client's perspective. The therapeutic work therefore involves not only tolerating the client's intense emotions, but tolerating the therapist's own intense emotions that may have been stirred up in the encounter. A clinical example of this process follows.

Example of Exploring Core Relational Themes (Expressive Repair Strategy)

CLIENT: Well, I'm not sure what to do here. I'm sort of stuck. My financial hole keeps getting deeper, I'm at the point where I don't have any money left at all. I don't know what I'm going to do to survive and it's scary. It's really scary.

THERAPIST: Why don't you try to talk to relatives and ask them for some financial help?

CLIENT: That's not going to work, they're not going to help me, I haven't talked to some of them in over 20 years.

THERAPIST: I see. Perhaps it would help if we set some goals here. Saying "I want my financial situation to be better" really isn't enough, and it's a difficult goal to operationalize. If you could distill that desire into a couple of concrete goals, what would they be?

CLIENT: I don't really know, it all just seems so hopeless. [Client becomes silent and despondent; Rupture Statement: Minimal responses from the client]

THERAPIST: What just happened there?

CLIENT: What do you mean?

THERAPIST: You became very quiet, I'm not sure where you went.

CLIENT: I don't know, it just all feels terrible. [Silence continues]

THERAPIST: I've been thinking about what's been happening in our sessions, and sometimes it feels to me like we're in a tug of war at times. I wonder if I'm doing something, too, that contributes to this push and pull. Do you have this experience? [Therapist Meta-communication: Therapist recognizes the rupture]

CLIENT: What do you mean?

THERAPIST: Just a moment ago, I was sort of pulling at you and trying to get you to come up with a financial goal, and it felt like you were pulling in the opposite direction. And shutting down, even.

CLIENT: I'm not sure what else to tell you; this is really hard for me to get out of. And I don't know what to do.

THERAPIST: Right, and I think I'm somewhat stuck, too, or rather, we're stuck here together with this. If either of us tries to move at all, we become more stuck. Do you see that? [Expressive Repair Strategy: Exploring core relational themes, therapist explores the rupture]

CLIENT: Yeah. [Silence] Yeah, I can get like that. It's hard for me to really get myself out of these things. [Expressive Repair Strategy: Exploring core relational themes, client also explores the rupture]

THERAPIST: Can you say more?

CLIENT: I think I'm just so tired of making mistakes; I feel like I've made so many. I just don't want to make any more. I would just rather have someone else make my decisions. I feel like I can't do it on my own. [Expressive Repair Strategy: Exploring core relational themes, client expresses a need]

THERAPIST: I wonder if this happens in here in other ways, too, meaning your wanting me to make your decisions for you.

CLIENT: What do you mean?

THERAPIST: Well, I found myself really compelled just now to give you advice to help fix your financial situation. Do you see that?

CLIENT: Yeah.

THERAPIST: But also, that advice wasn't what you were looking for, and you pushed back.

CLIENT: Yes.

THERAPIST: And we seem to get stuck in this, your wanting advice and then pushing back.

CLIENT: Yeah, I guess I see that.

In this example, the therapist attempts to understand the rupture that has occurred ("I've been thinking about what's been happening in our sessions, and sometimes it feels to me like we're in a tug of war at times. I wonder if I'm doing something, too, that contributes to this push and pull. Do you have this experience?"). The therapist and client then move toward exploration of the rupture process ("Right, and I think I'm somewhat stuck, too, or rather, we're stuck here together with this. If either of us tries to move at all, we become more stuck. Do you see that?"). Finally, the client moves toward an expression of need ("I would just rather have someone else make my decisions. I feel like I can't do it on my own"). This example illustrates the therapist's exploration of the rupture with the client while maintaining a stance of nonjudgmental curiosity throughout. The clinical maneuver that may be most difficult for novice clinicians is the task of staying in the rupture process with the client in an attempt to facilitate discussion about both the therapist's and client's experiences of the rupture; this can no doubt be a difficult undertaking due to management of the therapist's own emotions about the rupture encounter. It is not uncommon for therapists at all levels of training and expertise to find themselves feeling frustrated, inept, anxious, angry, and even hopeless when in the midst of a rupture. Novice clinicians may also find themselves questioning their skill and training or even may experience having their credentials questioned outright by their client. It is important for therapists to, as best as they can, attend to their own internal processes and emotions and open up an exploratory dialogue about the rupture with their client.

Summary

From our decades of research, we have found that addressing ruptures as they occur is a critical aspect of successful psychotherapy because therapists' abilities to recognize ruptures in their treatment has been linked to improved outcomes for clients along multiple symptom domains (Safran, Muran, & Eubanks-Carter, 2011). Ruptures can be organized into two categories: *withdrawal* and *confrontation* ruptures, and clients and therapists alike participate in these types of ruptures as they navigate their own conflicting needs of relatedness and agency. In repairing ruptures, our model makes use of the therapist's mindfulness skills in detecting the rupture, allowing the therapist to move toward addressing the rupture through immediate or expressive repair strategies. Expressive strategies make use of the skill of meta-communication in order to facilitate the therapist's exploration of the rupture. We hope that this guide will be a helpful primer in therapists' navigation of ruptures, an experience that is common in psychotherapy. Like many things in life, practice and continual learning will sharpen rupture repair strategies of novice and seasoned clinicians alike.

References

Anderson, T., McClintock, A. S., Himawan, L., Song, X., & Patterson, C. L. (2016). A prospective study of therapist facilitative interpersonal skills as a predictor of treatment outcome. *Journal of Consulting and Clinical Psychology, 84*(1), 57–66.

Aron, L. (1996). *Relational perspectives book series Vol. 4: A meeting of minds: Mutuality of psychoanalysis*. Mahwah, NJ: Analytic Press.

Aspland, H., Llewelyn, S., Hardy, G. E., Barkham, M., & Stiles, W. (2008). Alliance ruptures and rupture resolution in cognitive–behavior therapy: A preliminary task analysis. *Psychotherapy Research, 18*, 699–710.

Bambling, M., King, R., Raue, P., Schweittzer, R., & Lambert, W. (2006). Clinical supervision: Its influence on client-rated working alliance and client symptom reduction in the brief treatment of major depression. *Psychotherapy Research, 16*(3), 317–331.

Benjamin, J. (1990). An outline of intersubjectivity: The development of recognition. *Psychoanalytic Psychology, 7S*, 33–46.

Bennett, D., Parry, G., & Ryle, A. (2006). Resolving threats to the therapeutic alliance in cognitive analytic therapy of borderline personality disorder: A task analysis. *Psychology and Psychotherapy: Theory, Research, and Practice, 79*, 395–418.

Bordin, E. S. (1979). The generalizability of the psychoanalytic concept of the working alliance. *Psychotherapy: Theory, Research & Practice, 16*, 252–260.

The Boston Change Process Study Group. (2010). *Change in psychotherapy: A unifying paradigm*. New York: W. W. Norton & Co.

Crits-Christoph, P., Gibbons, M. B., Crits-Christoph, K., Narducci, J., Schamberger, M., & Gallop, R. (2006). Can therapists be trained to improve their alliances? A preliminary study of alliance-fostering psychotherapy. *Psychotherapy Research, 16*(3), 268–281.

Eubanks, C. F., Burckell, L. A., & Goldfried, M. R. (2018). Clinical consensus strategies to repair ruptures in the therapeutic alliance. *Journal of Psychotherapy Integration, 28*(1), 60–76.

Eubanks, C. F., Muran, J. C., & Safran, J. D. (2018). Alliance rupture repair: A meta-analysis. *Psychotherapy, 55*(4), 508–519.

Flückiger, C., Del Re, A. C., Wampold, B. E., Symonds, D., & Horvath, A. O. (2012). How central is the alliance in psychotherapy? A multilevel longitudinal meta-analysis. *Journal of Counseling Psychology, 59*(1), 10–17.

Freud, S. (1927). The Ego and the Id. In J. Strachey (Ed.), *The Standard Edition of the Complete Psychological Works of Sigmund Freud, Volume XIX (1923–1925): The Ego and the Id and Other Works* (pp. 1–66). London: Hogarth Press and Institute of Psycho-Analysis.

Harper, H. (1989a). *Coding Guide I: Identification of confrontation challenges in exploratory therapy*. Sheffield, UK: University of Sheffield Press.

Harper, H. (1989b). *Coding Guide II: Identification of withdrawal challenges in exploratory therapy*. Sheffield, UK: University of Sheffield Press.

Hill, C. E., Nutt-Williams, E., Heaton, K. J., Thompson, B. J., & Rhodes, R. H. (1996). Therapist retrospective recall impasses in long-term psychotherapy: A qualitative analysis. *Journal of Counseling Psychology, 43*(2), 207–217.

Horvath, A. O., & Greenberg, L. S. (1989). Development and validation of the Working Alliance Inventory. *Journal of Counseling Psychology, 36*(2), 223–233.

Horvath, A. O., & Symonds, B. D. (1991). Relation between working alliance and outcome in psychotherapy: A meta-analysis. *Journal of Counseling Psychology, 38*(2), 139–149.

Horvath, A. O., Del Re, A. C., Flückiger, C., & Symonds, D. (2011). Alliance in individual psychotherapy. *Psychotherapy, 48*(1), 9–16.

Jacobs, T. J. (1986). On countertransference enactments. *Journal of the American Psychoanalytic Association, 34*(2), 289–307.

Kiesler, D. J. (1996). *Contemporary interpersonal theory and research: Personality, psychopathology, and psychotherapy.* New York: Wiley.

Kohut, H. (1984). *How does analysis cure?* Chicago: University of Chicago Press.

Lambert, M. J. (2015). Progress feedback and the OQ-System: The past and the future. *Psychotherapy, 52*(4), 381–390.

Levendosky, A. A., & Hopwood, C. J. (2017). A clinical science approach to training first year clinicians to navigate therapeutic relationships. *Journal of Psychotherapy Integration, 27*(2), 153–171.

Luborsky, L. (1976). Helping alliances in psychotherapy. In J. L. Cleghhorn (Ed.), *Successful psychotherapy* (pp. 92–116). New York: Brunner/Mazel.

Martin, D. J., Garske, J. P., & Davis, M. K. (2000). Relation of the therapeutic alliance with outcome and other variables: Meta-analytic review. *Journal of Consulting & Clinical Psychology, 68*, 438–450.

Muran, J. C., & Eubanks, C. F. (in press). *Therapist performance under pressure: Negotiating emotion, difference and rupture.* Washington, DC: APA Books.

Muran, J. C., Samstag, L. W., Safran, J. D., & Winston, A. (2005). Evaluating an alliance-focused treatment for personality disorders. *Psychotherapy: Theory, Research, Practice, Training, 46*(2), 233–248.

Muran, J. C., Safran, J. D., & Eubanks-Carter, C. F. (2010). Developing therapist abilities to negotiate alliance ruptures. In J. C. Muran & J. P. Barber (Eds.), *The therapeutic alliance: An evidence-based guide to practice* (pp. 320–340). New York: Guilford Press.

Muran, J. C., Safran, J. D., Eubanks, C. F., & Gorman, B. S. (2018). The effect of alliance-focused training on a cognitive-behavioral therapy for personality disorders. *Journal of Consulting and Clinical Psychology, 86*(4), 384–397.

Safran, J. D., Crocker, P., McMain, S., & Murray, P. (1990). Therapeutic alliance rupture as a therapy event for empirical investigation. *Psychotherapy: Theory, Research, Practice, Training, 27*(2), 154–165.

Safran, J. D., & Muran, J. C. (1996). The resolution of ruptures in the therapeutic alliance. *Journal of Consulting and Clinical Psychology, 64*(3), 447–458.

Safran, J. D., & Muran, J. C. (2000). *Negotiating the therapeutic alliance: A relational treatment guide.* New York: Guilford Press.

Safran, J. D., Muran, J. C., Demaria, A, Boutwell, C, Eubanks-Carter, C. F., & Winston, A. (2014). Investigating the impact of alliance-focused training on interpersonal process and therapists' capacity for experiential reflection. *Psychotherapy Research, 24*(3), 269–285.

Safran, J. D., Muran, J. C., & Eubanks-Carter, C. (2011). Repairing alliance ruptures. *Psychotherapy, 48*(1), 80–87.

Safran, J. D., Muran, J. C., & Samstag, L. (1994). Resolving therapeutic alliance ruptures: A task analytic investigation. In A. O. Horvath & L. S. Greenberg (Eds.), *The working alliance: Theory, research and practice* (pp. 225–255). New York: Wiley.

Safran, J. D., Muran, J. C., Samstag, L. W., & Stevens, C. (2002). Repairing alliance ruptures. In J. C. Norcross (Ed.), *Psychotherapy relationships that work* (pp. 235–254). New York: Oxford University.

Stiles, W. B., Glick, M. J., Osatuke, K., Hardy, G. E., Shapiro, D. A., Agnew-Davies, R., . . . Barkham, M. (2004). Patterns of alliance development and the rupture-repair hypothesis: Are productive relationships U-shaped or V-shaped? *Journal of Counseling Psychology, 51*(1), 81–92.

9

Facilitating Supervisee Competence in Developing and Maintaining Working Alliances

Supervisor Roles and Strategies

Rodney Goodyear and Hideko Sera

The quality of the therapist–client working alliance predicts clients' persistence in treatment (Sharf, Primavera, & Diener, 2010) as well as the outcomes they achieve (Wampold & Imel, 2015). Therapist competence is a key variable in this process as more effective therapists are better able to establish strong alliances across a range of clients than are their less effective counterparts (Baldwin, Wampold, & Imel, 2007). This is true regardless of the model from which they work (see Flückiger, Del Re, Wampold, & Horvath, 2018). It is important, therefore, that training programs ensure that their graduates are able to develop and manage alliances with their clients. Supervisors are key to accomplishing this training goal.

At least a few studies have documented supervision's effects on the quality of the therapist–client alliance. Bambling, King, Raue, Schweitzer, and Lambert (2006) found that when experienced therapists were randomly assigned to one of two types of supervision or to a no-supervision condition, those who received either form of supervision had stronger alliances with their clients than those in the no-supervision condition. Patton and Kivlighan (1997) had earlier found that the quality of the supervisee–client alliance varied in accordance with the quality of the supervisory alliance. Both studies were important in having documented that supervision can affect the supervisee–client alliance. But no study of which we are aware has examined whether supervision effects endure or, more importantly, translate to increased therapist competence in alliance development and maintenance.

In fact, with only a few exceptions (e.g., Eubanks-Carter, Muran, & Safran, 2015), the literature has provided supervisors with little guidance about how to help supervisees develop this competence. Our purpose in writing this chapter is to add to that small literature by discussing strategies supervisors can employ to help trainees develop competence in alliance development and maintenance. In the first section of the chapter, we address supervisor instructional practices that do not *specifically* target the supervisee–client alliance, but which are important to that purpose. In the second chapter, we discuss areas of supervisor focus that directly or indirectly improve supervisees' competence in alliance development and maintenance.

Supervisor Instructional Practices

The four instructional strategies we discuss are essential in fostering many supervisee competencies, including those related to alliance development and maintenance. The first three—the use of video in supervision, the use of routine outcome monitoring, and supervisor modeling—are essential to any good supervision. The fourth, deliberate practice, is an emerging supervision technology that has a great deal of promise for developing alliance-related competencies.

Video-Informed Feedback in Supervision

Haggerty and Hilsenroth (2011) asked readers to imagine that a loved one who is about to undergo surgery has a choice between two new surgeons: one learned surgery by conducting surgery and then returning to her supervisor to report as carefully as possible exactly what she had done, whereas the other surgeon had learned by having a supervisor who directly observed and coached. The choice, of course, is clear. But whereas no reputable training program would teach surgeons on the basis of their self-reports, that is not at all the case in psychology training. Self-report remains the most frequently used modality in the supervision of novice psychotherapists (Amerikaner & Rose, 2012; Borders, Cashwell, & Rotter, 1995).

No retrospective verbal description can capture the complex interpersonal behaviors that occur between therapist and client. In fact, Wynne, Susman, Ries, Birringer, and Katz (1994) found that licensed psychologists were able to recall molar (i.e., main) and molecular (i.e., supporting) ideas from therapy sessions at rates of only 42% and 30%, respectively. Earlier, Muslin, Thurnblad, and Meschel (1981) had found that supervisees reported less than half of the issues that supervisors found important when reviewing their videos. But these difficulties in reporting are compounded by the fact that almost all supervisees intentionally withhold (Knox, 2015) or distort (Yourman & Farber, 1996) information they provide their supervisors.

In short, self-report has substantial limitations as a supervision modality, despite its near-universal use. These limitations are sufficiently problematic considering that American Psychological Association's (APA) supervision standards (APA, 2015) now state that supervisors are expected to directly observe at least some of their supervisees' work, and Ellis et al. (2014) asserted that doing so is a necessary element of minimally competent supervision. Direct observation can include live observation, co-therapy with the supervisee, or video recordings, each of which has advantages. But video review is especially valuable in enabling the supervisor and supervisee to very closely analyze supervisee–client interaction sequences.

To speak more directly, then, to the purpose of this chapter: video review is essential to helping supervisees develop competence in alliance building and maintenance. It enables supervisors to help supervisees address processes that directly affect the alliance, such as developing the skills to offer a convincing treatment rationale or to identify interpersonal patterns that suggest that the alliance needs attention. But, as well, supervisee competence in areas such as managing countertransference also will affect that quality of the alliance, and video review is essential there as well.

Finally, we would observe that there is no one way to use video in supervision. Supervisors can make choices about the use of recording devices according to the supervisee's needs and their training goals. For example, supervisors might observe a video with the supervisee and then provide feedback and direct instruction about relational behaviors that would improve the alliance. Alternatively, they can use video to encourage self-discovery and reflection by using such strategies as Interpersonal Process Recall (Kagan & Kagan, 1990). But the strength in any use of video is the opportunity it affords supervisor and supervisee to catch and address very specific behaviors and interactions.

Using Routine Outcome Monitoring in Supervision

It would be unusual for a visit to a physician's office not to begin with a check on the patient's pulse rate, temperature, and blood pressure. This is an expected standard of care. But monitoring their clients' "vital signs" is still relatively new to therapists. In fact, it has been only a couple of decades since Howard, Moras, Brill, Martinovich, and Lutz (1996) argued that the profession should adopt routine session-by-session monitoring as an expectation. The Outcome Questionnaire (OQ)-45 (Lambert, 2015) quickly became the dominant means for that monitoring, followed then by a now-burgeoning number of additional routine outcome monitoring (ROM) tools (see Boswell, Kraus, Miller, & Lambert, 2015).

Using ROM data is now understood to be a central aspect of evidence-based practice (APA, 2006).

The "vital signs" with which therapists should be concerned include both clients' progress (as measured by week-to-week changes in their functioning) and the client's perception of the quality of the therapist–client alliance. However, some ROM measures have included only measures of client progress. This was true, for example, of the OQ-45, though later a companion measure was developed to assess alliance and other factors (Lambert, 2015). Other systems, especially the Partners for Change Outcome Management System (PCOMS; Miller, Duncan, Sorrell, & Brown, 2005), have included *both* client progress and alliance measures (the PCOMS measures also have the advantage of brevity as the client progress and the alliance measures each have only four items).

ROM feedback about both client progress and the alliance are invaluable to supervision (see, e.g., Swift et al., 2015). Client feedback allows the supervisor and supervisee to better detect when clients are not progressing as expected or when the client is rating the alliance lower than expected and then to identify both the problem and solutions (this does not, of course, substitute for supervisee–client conversations about their relationship, which supervisees should be having in any case).

Video review is an especially useful option when ROM data signal a significant fluctuation in the supervisee–client alliance as it permits the supervisor and supervisee to review interaction events and patterns. In reviewing a video of a session in which the fluctuation is *positive*, the supervisee has the potential to learn something important that might generalize to work with other clients. The same, of course, is true if the fluctuation is *negative* as it allows the supervisor and supervisee to identify possible changes in how the supervisee is working with the client; in some cases, it might suggest new skills for the supervisee to learn. Once that has occurred, continuing video review of work with that client can help monitor subsequent sessions in order to continue to fine-tune responses, thus strengthening the supervisee's alliance-related competence.

Teaching by Example: The Importance of Modeling

The notion that there is an important correspondence between events in counselor supervision and counseling suggests that interpersonal interactions in supervision should have an impact on such elements of the counseling process as the working alliance.

—Patton & Kivilighan (1997, p. 108)

One of the more illuminating discoveries for novice trainees concerns the extent to which their interactions with their clients often have a parallel in other interpersonal contexts, including in their supervision. In speaking of this, Patton and Kivlighan (1997) were addressing a correspondence of *events*. But, as well, there are fundamental structural similarities (i.e., isomorphism) between supervision and therapy, and these contribute to supervision-to-therapy or therapy-to-supervision transmission mechanisms, such as parallel processes (White & Russell, 1997). *Supervisor modeling*, another of those transmission mechanisms, is particularly important as it accounts for enduring effects rather than transient processes. Those effects include supervisees' values and theoretical models (Guest & Beutler, 1988), professionalism (Price, Roberts, Fatollahi, & Gandhi, 2016), technical skills (Goodyear, 2014), and, of course, alliance-related competencies.

Supervisors' opportunities to teach through example begin with the very first supervision session. It occurs, for example, as the supervisor and supervisee collaborate to develop a supervision contract, now an expected supervisor practice (APA, 2015). Developing this contract should include a process of discussing the supervisor's and supervisee's mutual responsibilities and their expectations for each other (Bernard & Goodyear, 2019), including the goals for that work and how they will accomplish those goals. This is a direct analogue to the important alliance-related processes in therapy of establishing goals and tasks. It might be useful, in fact, to make that parallel explicit.

This contracting process also should include discussions the supervisor and supervisee have about their differences (e.g., power dynamics that emerge in gender, race or ethnicity, age, and so on), how those differences may affect their work together, and the importance of mutual permission to address any issues that might seem to emerge from those differences. Similarly, the contracting process should include a discussion of how supervisor and supervisee will address conflict and relationship strains or ruptures more broadly. These conversations provide supervisees with a model for similar conversations that they should have with their clients.

But, regardless of supervisors' intent to teach at any given moment, supervisees continuously learn from what they observe of their supervisors' behavior. In some cases, unfortunately, supervisees will learn what *not* to do. For example, supervisees are both affected by and learn from how the supervisor respects boundaries between them, how the supervisor models humility, how the supervisor makes it safe to discuss relationship strains, and how the supervisor embodies particular interventions or interpersonal behaviors. Erving Polster demonstrated the last of these effectively in his supervision in Goodyear's (1982) video series, employing immediacy and genuineness with the supervisee—qualities that had been lacking in the supervisee's interactions with his client. In so doing, Polster taught by example.

In summary, supervisees always are learning from what they observe about their supervisors. This speaks to the importance of attending to the quality of the supervisory alliance on an ongoing basis, both for its immediate benefits in supervision and for what it is teaching supervisees about their own relationships with clients.

Deliberate Practice

Ericsson, Krampe, and Tesch-Römer (1993) found that violin and piano students who achieved the highest career goals (e.g., became performance artists) spent *many* more hours in practice than their less accomplished peers who, for example, taught others or only continued playing as a hobby. Gladwell (2008) popularized the Ericsson et al. finding as the "10,000 hour rule": that it takes 10,000 hours of practice to become an expert in any domain. Although this is oversimplified, it makes the important point that developing expertise requires extensive practice. Gladwell also employed examples (e.g., the Beatles playing thousands of hours in performances) that seemed to miss the essential point that expertise is not developed simply by engaging in extensive amounts of work-as-usual. Were that the case, psychotherapists would improve with experience, but most do not (Goldberg, Rousmaniere, et al., 2016).

Ericsson et al. (1993) believed that the key was *deliberate practice* (DP) that supplemented ordinary work activities. In fact, Chow and his colleagues (2015) validated the importance of DP for therapists. They found that therapists who were in the top quartile in terms of client outcomes spent twice as much time in DP activities as those in the second quartile and four times as much as those in the bottom quartile. Goldberg, Babins-Wagner, et al. (2016) also were able to document the importance of DP in their study of one counseling center that had systematically adopted DP as an organization expectation: in this case, therapists actually did become more effective across time as one of the rare exceptions to the general rule that therapists do not improve with time.

Miller, Hubble, and Chow (2017) describe DP in psychotherapy as having four elements: (1) focused, systematic, and ongoing efforts to improve performance; (2) supervision or consultation to guide those efforts; (3) continual feedback (from supervisor or consultant; from supervisees and consultees); and (4) continual solo practice outside of performance to refine professional practice. It is "a highly structured activity, the explicit goal of which is to improve performance" (Ericsson et al., 1993, p. 368). The last of the Miller et al. conditions—solo practice outside of what one regularly does in practice—is probably the element that most sets it apart from usual supervision practices.

To give an example of how a supervisor might use DP to build alliance-related competence, we list the following:

1. The supervisor and supervisee would identify and review a video recording (perhaps chosen on the basis of ROM feedback) to identify an event or sequence that relates to some specific aspect of alliance development or maintenance that the supervisee might improve.
2. They might then agree on how the supervisees' work might be improved, and the supervisor would help the supervisee identify several alternative responses that she or he could have made during the session.
3. The supervisee would be assigned to set aside a block of time (perhaps 20 minutes) several times during the coming week to view a specified section of that video and practice delivering those alternative responses, saying them aloud multiple times to the computer screen as she or he watches the video.

This supervisor approach to DP derives from Tony Rousmaniere's (see https://www.dpfortherapists.com/) work. But the use of DP is still very new, and a number of people (e.g., Daryl Chow, Scott Miller, and Bruce Wampold) now are involved in developing DP strategies that supervisors should have available to them soon.

Earlier in the chapter, we discussed the use of video review in supervision. Supervisors can obtain excellent guidance in knowing *what* to attend to in those reviews by using Chow and Miller's (Chow et al., 2015) *Taxonomy of Deliberate Practice Activities* to guide DP in supervision (parallel forms for supervisors and therapists). One of the *Taxonomy*'s five sections explicitly focuses on developing alliance-related skills, which are broken into four components, each with specific goals for supervisees. These components are "Effective Focus" (e.g., How do you help a client who has no clear goals in therapy?), "The Impact Factor" (e.g., How do you explicitly convey empathic attunement?), "Motivation" (e.g., How do you assess and work with a client's motivation to change?), and "Difficulties" (e.g., How do you deal with alliance rupture?). Miller makes the *Taxonomy* available for free (https://scott-d-miller-ph-d.myshopify.com/collections/performance-metrics/products/performance-metrics-licenses-for-the-ors-and-srs) for those who register (also free) for the Outcome Rating and Session Rating Scale because he considers using those scales to be the first step in determining a supervisee's baseline (see the earlier discussion about ROM in supervision).

Supervision Focus

Many client, therapist, and contextual factors can affect the quality of therapeutic alliances. For example, both clients and therapists bring relationship histories and expectations that affect the quality and strength of the therapeutic alliance (e.g., Hersoug, Monsen, Havik, & Høglend, 2002), and Anderson and his colleagues (Anderson, Crowley, Himawan, Holmberg, & Uhlin, 2016) have identified measurable therapist interpersonal qualities such as verbal fluency and persuasiveness that predict client outcomes and client ratings of alliance but which are relatively resistant to training. Although supervisors should not ignore those supervisee qualities, they are probably best attended to when applicants are being screened into training programs.

Fortunately, supervision can have useful effects by focusing on particular attitudinal and skill-related issues that bear on alliance-related competence. In Chapter 8, Muran and colleagues speak to strategies in addressing fluctuations in the alliance. This chapter complements their work by focusing on supervisor strategies intended to help supervisees develop broader competencies related to alliance development and maintenance. In the sections that follow, we will address multicultural competence, focusing on technique at the expense of relationship, establishing a treatment rationale, skills in "meta-communicating," developing competence in recognizing alliance strains and ruptures, managing countertransference, and developing self-care competencies.

Fostering Multicultural Competence to Foster Alliance-Related Competence

Supervisees' ability to manage complex issues such as gender, race, class, age, language, sexual orientation, religions, abilities, and many other social issues affects how well they will develop and maintain alliances with their clients. This means that supervision must have an ongoing focus on helping supervisees develop multicultural competencies if they are to be successful in developing and maintaining alliances with their clients.

The demographics of both the profession and the clients it serves are changing. For instance, there are more ethnoracially diverse early career psychologists than a few decades ago, despite the continuing dominance of non-Hispanic white psychologists (http://www.apa.org/workforce/presentations/convention-symposium.pdf: APA—report on demographics). There are also multicultural differences in treatment-seeking behaviors (Alegría et al., 2008; Gallo, Marino, Ford, & Anthony, 1995) and in the people who seek treatment. For example, all five of the states with the largest numbers of active psychologists (California, New York, Illinois, Florida, and Texas) are characterized by substantially increasing diversity with respect to ethnicity, race, country of origin, and languages other than English spoken, especially at home. Therapists who are not competent in working with these populations will have difficulties in navigating through various challenges that complex and diverse situations present in therapeutic settings.

The supervision's multicultural literature has mostly ignored context in communication (Gudykunst & Nishida, 1986). Specifically, *high-context cultures*, which primarily are those that are more collectivist, rely on communication that is nuanced and for which meaning is implicit in the participant's interactions, whereas *low-context cultures* rely on messaging that is more explicit, verbal, and intentional. Park and Kim (2008) noted, for example, that people employing a high-context style will be more prone to using silence, to inferring the meaning of the other person's messages, and to relying on their feelings to guide their interactions, whereas those employing a low-context style will be more animated, friendly, open, dramatic, dominant, and contentious. These high- versus low-context differences are reflected, for example, in how the parties in a relationship will attempt to resolve conflict (Croucher et al., 2012), which is key to alliance maintenance. Supervisees need to learn to identify indicators of alliance ruptures that may be affected by culture. For example, the extent to which the client relies on high- versus low-context communication may determine how she or he conveys relationship problems. Supervisors can play an especially important role in helping supervisees to identify those cues. This, of course, requires that supervisors are themselves developing and maintaining their own multicultural competence (see APA, 2015). The following case vignette highlights how supervisors might discuss diversity factors that are influencing supervisees and their clients.

Maria is a quiet and shy Mexican American doctoral student who began seeing a Mexican American female client with anxiety symptoms a few weeks ago. Maria believes one reason her client is experiencing anxiety is due to her relationship with her boyfriend who is unhappy with her recent job promotions. In their therapy, Maria's client reports that her Mexican American boyfriend does not like the fact she now earns more money than him and indicates that it makes her "very nervous" that her boyfriend makes demeaning and sniping comments when they are out with other couples (e.g., that she is developing extravagant tastes now that she is making "so much money"). She also adds that her boyfriend hints that he does not know of any other couples where women are making more money than men. Maria senses that her client has suppressed her frustration and uses therapy as a way to release it. Coupled with her quiet temperament, Maria lets her client to vocalize her frustration and anger.

A few weeks into therapy, Maria's client directly asks Maria why she is so quiet. "Why are you not like me? We are from the same culture, and why are you so quiet? Why are you not really saying anything? Why are you so different from me? Is this because you are more educated?" Maria is surprised by this confrontation because she genuinely believes that she has been helping her client release her frustration by letting her speak uninterrupted. Maria believed she's taken a truly client-centered approach and had thought treatment was going well.

In supervision, Maria brings up her surprise at her client's emotional reaction. Her supervisor, an Italian American from Brooklyn, begins by disclosing how he was always seen as an outlier in his community as someone who grew up extremely quiet and shy. He then talks about cultural expectations that everyone faces, regardless of their backgrounds, and how they are amplified at times in therapeutic relationships. Maria self-reflectively shares with her supervisor that the most surprising element of her client's confrontation was her accusation and expectation that she and Maria are not similar and that it could be due to educational differences. Maria adds that she has always expected clients from other backgrounds to have difficulties with her, but never expected difficulties with someone who comes from the same background. This leads Maria's supervisor to urge Maria to notice similarities and differences between her and her client, as her client did so, and how they are impacting therapeutic alliance. Specifically, Maria's supervisor asks the following questions:

1. When your client pointed out the differences between you and her, what do you think she was trying to communicate? What do you think your client wanted from you at that moment?
2. What experiences have you had as an outlier in your own cultural upbringing and environment? What strengths and challenges did you experience because you were different?
3. Although you are reporting that your client's expectation for you two to be similar was upsetting, you have also indicated you never expected such confrontations to come from people who share your cultural background. Let's talk about the duality of this. As your client expected you not to be different from her, you have also expected people from your cultural background to not have difficulties with you.
4. Let's talk about the symbolism of education and educated people in your culture. What does that mean? What is the cost of becoming a well-educated Mexican American woman? How is that similar or different

from a well-paid Mexican American woman? What are differences and similarities between you and your client?

5. Often when we are not getting what we want from another person, we act in a way that pressures the other person to give us what we want. Are there ways in which your client is asking you to give her something she needs that you are not picking up?

Over the course of few weeks, although at times emotionally overwhelming, Maria and her supervisor address these questions. Maria's deep and self-reflective process then leads to a few realizations that drastically change her therapeutic relationship with her client. Specifically, Maria and her client engage in dialogues that elicit honest and authentic interactions about their similarities and differences. Maria also realizes that when her client became confrontational, she really was asking Maria to validate her, that she was not alone in her pursuit of having more confidence and less guilt for the fact she's more financially powerful than her boyfriend.

Often, when multiculturalism is discussed in literature, it focuses on respect and appreciation toward diversity. What we propose specifically here is that diversity is an essential component of every relationship—therapeutic ones included. As no one person is alike, with his or her complex cultural experiences that shape expectations and experiences of self and others, every therapeutic process is an opportunity for supervisors to attend to the intersection of colliding or overlapping worldviews of supervisees and their clients while they also attend to how their *own* worldviews affect their supervision styles. Ackerman and Hilsenroth (2001) observed that "the interaction between the patient and therapist is impacted by the values, beliefs, relational patterns, and expectations each participant brings into the treatment room" (p. 172). It is also important for supervisors to note that perceived similarity to the client with respect to such characteristics as ethnoracial status can lend the therapist credibility (see, e.g., Raven, 2008 for a review of the model behind this assertion), and, for this reason, supervisees need to be mindful of how their clients react toward them and their therapeutic alliance builds. Specifically, there are times when clients are eager to build connections simply due to the perceived similarities between them and their therapists. Conversations related to multicultural factors in therapeutic and/or supervisory relationships can provoke discomfort. But it is in these moments that supervisors model cultural humility and self-reflectiveness. Specifically, supervisors could promote asking such questions as:

1. Whenever we talk about differences between you and your client, I have observed that you tense up. If I am observing this tendency, what do you think your client is able to pick up as well?
2. How do you believe your own beliefs about self, others, and world impact your client's beliefs?
3. Although multiculturalism and diversity issues may not become the center of every therapeutic relationship and session, it is important for us (in supervision) to always discuss how these issues impact your relationships with your clients. What honest reactions do you experience when working with people who hold similar values to yours? What happens when you work with people who hold different values? What happens when you work with people whose ideas and values are, in your eyes, despicable? What do you need to overcome these reactions, because you are expected to deliver consistent care to all people who seek your help?

At the core of these difficult but necessary dialogues in supervision about diversity is trust-building: trust is essential to alliance development, and many training programs provide an intellectual basis for multicultural competence in research, treatment, and policies while practicum and internship experiences provide an opportunity to improve therapeutic skills related to diversity. However, what is often the most challenging is indeed in the area of one's values and attitudes that impact elements essential to alliance, such as trust, authenticity, respect, and reflective skills. For this reason, it is the supervisor who helps develop this last component in practice.

Substantive, meaningful, and thoughtful diversity dialogues that respectfully address differences and their impact on our relational dynamics do not easily come to most people, and many supervisees would benefit from direct observation of how their supervisors engage in these dialogues with them. Through struggling and at times uncomfortable dialogues between supervisors and supervisees about their differences and sameness, supervisors may earn trust from supervisees to continue deepening these dialogues. And, in turn, supervisees not only directly observe but also experience what the alliance-building process feels like, to them, in a dyad.

Earlier in the chapter we noted the importance of ROM for teaching alliance-related competence. Swift et al. (2015) have discussed one means of using those data to identify possible multicultural challenges for the supervisee. This involves summarizing client ROM data on a spreadsheet, with mean scores for each client, who also is identified by ethnoracial or gender categories. If a review of those data were to show that clients of a particular ethnoracial group rated the supervisee's alliance with them as lower than for other groups, the supervision could focus on possible causes and remedies.

Balancing Focus on Treatment Technique with Attention to the Alliance

Therapists often will retain vivid memories of a particular supervisor's behaviors or statements, even years later (Geller, Farber, & Schaffer, 2010). One of us (HS) has a number of those memories from work with her supervisor, the late Harold Mosak. She particularly remembers his caution to "not decide too early" about interventions. Mosak understood how supervisees often will too eagerly implement techniques or treatment protocols without having fully understood their clients' needs or having obtained the client's buy-in. This comes at the expense, however, of therapist–client agreement on tasks and goals, both of which are essential to an effective alliance (Bordin, 1979).

Some of this occurs from supervisees' eagerness to learn and to try out their newly developing skills. Supervisees' wish to impress their supervisors with their technical competence is another, nontrivial factor. For those and other reasons, it can be normative for novice therapists to overly focus on technical adherence to a model to the possible detriment of the therapist–client alliance (e.g., Stoltenberg, Bailey, Cruzan, Hart, & Ukuku, 2014). But although more experienced therapists may be less prone to this, there are circumstances in which their focus on technique can negatively affect their alliances with clients. For example, Henry, Strupp, Butler, Schacht, and Binder (1993) found that therapists who were being trained in a new model (time-limited dynamic therapy) experienced some relationship deterioration with their clients. This might also happen when therapists are attending to "doing it right" with respect to their model while neglecting the alliance, as Castonguay, Goldfried, Wiser, Raue, and Hayes (1996) found with cognitive therapists.

The challenge for supervisors is how to relieve supervisees from feeling so pressured to perform technically that they do not attend sufficiently to authentic relational interactions with their clients. One approach supervisors might take is educative: familiarizing supervisees with the literature showing that technical skills account for less variance in therapy outcomes than do relational skills (see Wampold & Imel, 2015) and with the compelling work of Anderson and colleagues that shows that what they call *facilitative interpersonal skills* are robustly predictive of therapy outcomes (see Anderson, McClintock, Himawan, Song, & Patterson, 2016; and Chapter 3). But having this information alone is unlikely to suffice by itself: in our experience, new supervisees come to believe in the power of the therapy relationship only as they gain experience and as their supervisors allow them to discover this without the pressure to perform technically.

It is important that supervisees learn to implement a model of treatment. Indeed, the supervisee's ability to enlist the client in a shared understanding of what they will be doing together and to what ends is essential to alliance formation and maintenance (as we discuss in the section that follows). Supervisors therefore should help supervisees adhere to model-specified skills *but* while also helping them be attentive and responsive to cues related to alliance strength and quality. The result of those stronger alliances should be better client outcomes than when fidelity-to-model has precedence (see Owen & Hilsenroth, 2014).

Bob is a new therapist who is now midway through his first practicum. Ann, his supervisor, has become concerned about the extent to which she finds herself pulled into the role of teacher, giving Bob technical instruction on his skills. She recognizes that focusing to this extent on skill development is not unusual for someone at his level. But Bob's level of skills is consistent with someone at his level of experience, and she observes that focusing on skills is coming at the expense of his relationship quality with his clients. She offers Bob this feedback, and they agree then to allocate a portion of each session to the use of Interpersonal Process Recall (IPR; Kagan & Kagan, 1990).

In each session, they discuss the video(s) Bob has brought and agree on the segment that would be most useful to review. Following IPR protocol, Bob is to play the video and stop it whenever anything at all occurs to him. Ann's role is simply to ask questions that will help Bob reflect on himself and his therapy: during their IPR work she offers no reflections or interpretations and certainly no teaching.

Ann chooses questions that will help him become both more self-aware (e.g., "What did you feel like doing?" "Do you remember what you were feeling?" "Did you fantasize any risks?") and the quality of his relationships with clients (e.g., "What did you think she or he was feeling about you?" "Did you feel that he or she had any expectations of you at that point?" "Did you want her or him to see you in some particular way?" "How?" "Was there anything in particular you wanted her or him to say or do or think?" "Is that the image you wanted to project?").

As their work progresses, Ann observes that Bob's alliances with his clients seem to be improving. She also notices that it has changed the work they are doing in the portions of their supervision sessions that do not involve IPR because the material Bob presents is less about skills and more about the quality of his relationships with his clients.

Establishing a Treatment Rationale

Muran et al. (Muran, Safran, & Eubanks-Carter, 2011) observed that the field often has given too little emphasis to therapists being able to convey an explicit and compelling treatment rationale to their clients. Supervisors, too, have often overlooked this as a competence their supervisees are to develop. Yet both Wampold's (2017) contextual model and the earlier Frank and Frank (1993) model both emphasized how important it is that (a) the therapist is able to provide the client with a conceptual scheme (or, "myth") that explains how the client's problems developed and describes procedures or rituals that will be used to ameliorate those problems and that (b) the client finds both the myth and associated rituals convincing. Sue and Zane (2009), in discussing multicultural therapy, describe the provided rationale as an instance of "giving" or providing the client with the sense that she or he has received something from the therapist.

> Explanations of treatment are intended to provide a rationale and to alter clients' expectations so that they fit the therapy process. In other words, we attempt to change their expectations to match our form of treatment. Such a strategy is needed in order to deal with clients who do not understand the treatment process. (p. 9)

This is an important process in establishing trust, as well the agreement and collaboration on goals and tasks that are crucial to the alliance (Bordin, 1979).

Being able to provide a compelling rationale or explanation requires that supervisees are sufficiently clear about their treatment model so that they can be effective in describing its assumptions and treatment methods. That level of clarity is probably higher for students in training programs that are explicit about teaching a particular model than for students in programs that give them latitude to "discover" what model fits best for them. But developing clarity about their model is important for all supervisees and therefore an important focus in supervision.

Providing a compelling rationale is only part of the process. In the spirit of establishing consensus and collaboration that underlies the alliance, supervisees must also know how to elicit the client's understandings of the origins or nature of their problem and how the client thinks that the problem can be "fixed." For example, if the supervisee who is operating from a cognitive-behavioral therapy model works with a client who explains his or her problems in terms of punishment from God for having committed some serious sin, it would be important to know that very early in the treatment. This gives both the supervisor and supervisee important information and the opportunity to strategize and find ways for the supervisee to find common ground with the client with respect to the goals and tasks of treatment.

There are two circumstances in which it is important for supervisors to be able to help supervisees convey their treatment rationales to clients: in the supervisee's initial sessions with the client when they are developing their alliance and expectations for one another, and then later, as relationship strains or ruptures might emerge that seem to concern in some way the rationale and goals of their work together. Supervisors may find it helpful in these tasks to draw from the chapters in Barlow's (2014) edited book that discuss how therapists might provide treatment rationales to clients, or from Ermold, Lefkowitz, and Santanello's (n.d.) tips about that process.

With respect to the first circumstance—the initial stages of alliance development—the supervisor should help the supervisee be able to:

1. Deliver the treatment rationale in a simple, conversational way. The advantage to helping the supervisee develop and deliver that rationale is that it requires the supervisee be able to articulate the model from which she or he is working—which may still be developing and only implicit.
2. Use this as an opportunity to discuss with clients their own beliefs and expectations about both the nature of their problems and of therapy.
3. Understand that clients are often anxious or otherwise distracted in their first session and so they may encode only portions of this discussion. The supervisee should be prepared then to have this as a conversation that will continue. It also could help to have the client summarize his or her understandings of the rationale after having discussed it with the therapist.

The second circumstance in which treatment rationale can come up as a supervision focus can occur when a relationship strain or rupture between the supervisee and his or her client has occurred. In the section that immediately follows, we discuss meta-communication or immediacy as a means to address the rupture. It is possible that the rupture occurred because of some supervisee–client interpersonal dynamic (e.g., that the supervisee has responded insensitively or otherwise had "missed" what the client was needing). But, in other cases, the client's shaken belief in the treatment and its effects are at the root of the rupture. In those instances, the supervisor can help the supervisee revisit the rationale and goals, being prepared to be responsive to the client's doubts or concerns.

Skills in Meta-Communicating

Meta-communication, or being able to discuss therapist–client communications with each other (Kiesler, 1988; Watzlawick, Beavin, & Jackson, 1967), is important across a range of situations in therapy. But it is especially valuable in resolving relationship impasses, strains, and ruptures (e.g., Eubanks-Carter et al., 2015; Hill & Knox, 2009; Muran et al., 2011). By meta-communicating, the therapist is able to make manifest interaction patterns that would otherwise go unacknowledged, making it possible to focus on and resolve those that are problematic.

Meta-communication, also called *immediacy* (Hill & Knox, 2009), is easier for some supervisees to master than others. There is a skill component to it. But, as well, this intervention invites the client to engage with the therapist in a "real" relationship (see Gelso, 2014) that requires more than simple mastery of technique. Immediacy has positive effects on clients' perception of their therapy (Hill et al., 2014; Shafran, Kivlighan, Gelso, Bhatia, & Hill, 2017). There are different types of immediacy interventions (Hill, 2014), and Hill et al. (2014) found that some therapists used immediacy to focus on feelings and not on alliance ruptures. Immediacy used to focus on ruptures may occur when the supervisee senses that the client has been particularly disengaged over the past couple of sessions. This is an invitation to address a possible rupture with the client, and the supervisee should be prepared to process the client's reactions to the use of immediacy (e.g., an expression of disappointment with the progress of therapy—or perhaps with the therapist as well) nondefensively and as helpfully as possible. This can be difficult, particularly for a supervisee, but it is essential to alliance formation or repair. Supervisors can play an important role in helping supervisees to use immediacy. For example,

- *To recognize markers for the use of rupture-focused immediacy*: this will be clearer with confrontive client behavior but can be less so for withdrawal behaviors (which we address more explicitly in the next section).
- *To navigate the challenging situations that can then result with the use of immediacy.* Some of these can occur by eliciting the supervisee's review and reflection about what occurred or, perhaps better, review and discussion of a video recording of one of those difficult interpersonal sequences. But it also is important that supervisors be willing to model effective meta-communication with their supervisees.

Consider the following scenario.

Mary, a supervisor in a university counseling center, is working with David, a doctoral student in counseling who is completing an externship at the counseling center. David is working with a student who had presented with depression and initially had been quite engaged in her therapy. But this has changed, and, in their most recent session, she not only actively resists several of David's statements but mentions how helpful her previous therapist had been. In reviewing the video recording of this session, Mary and David discuss how he might address this process between them.

But given the several times the client had actively "pushed back" on David's interventions in their most recent session, he is anxious both about how she might respond if he were to meta-communicate about what seems to be occurring between them and about how he will be able to remain helpful in his response, in turn, to her response. To help him prepare, Mary has David rehearse, using role-plays in which she takes the role of the client and enacts several possible client responses. She also recognizes how useful modeling can be in teaching immediacy and so finds an opportunity to comment on their relationship and then processes with him.

As they rehearse in this way, David not only builds more confidence in his eventual handling of the relationship rupture but gains more empathy for his client and her experiences. As well, Mary's use of immediacy concerning their own relationship afforded him the opportunity to observe her delivery of the response as well as the resulting effects on their own interactions: both are important lessons for his intervention with his client.

Developing Competence in Recognizing Alliance Strains and Ruptures

In complex therapeutic relationships supervisees are able to identify some problems, while others are difficult to identify and manage. Muran et al. (2011) observe that relationship ruptures tend to be marked by one of two kinds of behaviors: client *withdrawal* and client *confrontation*. In many cases the latter behaviors are more obvious, though even they can be difficult, as for example, when they are manifest as being overly friendly.

We stress the importance of directly observing the supervisees' work to help them identify relation strains that may not be apparent to them. This direct observation also promotes the supervisor to encourage the supervisee to have regular conversations with their clients about how they are perceiving their treatment. For instance, it is helpful for supervisors to inform supervisees that, in their ongoing supervision sessions, supervisees reporting back direct treatment feedback from clients is an integral part of every supervision session. Supervisors viewing and reviewing the exact segment of therapy when their supervisees are asking for treatment feedback from their clients is, therefore, a critical element of supervision.

The following vignette illustrates some of these processes and highlights how supervisors may approach supervisees' alliance rupture and strains with their clients.

During her advanced practicum, Susan was assigned to work with a client with substantial trust issues resulting from early traumatic relational difficulties. In their 8 weeks of work together, Susan's client would either shut down, sometimes with apathetic expressions and other times with rage, or verbally attack Susan for not knowing what to do to alleviate her emotional pain. Susan, new to managing the level of emotional inconsistencies her client exhibited, approaches her supervisor for guidance.

Observing video recordings of Susan's work, her supervisor realizes that Susan, too, shuts down when her client withdraws from therapeutic dynamic. Based on these reviews, Susan's supervisor realizes that Susan and her client actually are mirroring each other's emotional dynamics, especially in the way that Susan follows her client's lead of emotional withdrawals and attacks in therapy. Susan's supervisor decides to ask her a few questions to guide her reflection on her sessions. Specifically, the supervisor asks (1) how Susan is obtaining systematic and ongoing information about her client's impressions about therapeutic progress, (2) what interaction patterns lead Susan's client to emotionally withdraw from therapy, and (3) why Susan's client has continued to participate in therapy for eight sessions although she withdraws or lashes out at Susan at times.

Susan shares with her supervisor that she is afraid of asking her client for her impressions of therapeutic progress, and indeed this is the client she dreads seeing every week. She also recognizes that she is frightened by both her client's rejection and her expression of raw emotions. Susan then realizes that her client must be getting something out of therapy, although it often feels broken, and she decides to ask her client directly about what it is that she is getting out of the relationship. Susan's client breaks down and says that she has been "testing" Susan's patience, and the reason why she returns for her weekly session with Susan is because she does not give up on her.

Susan also realizes that the reason why she tries to contain the session is because she does not want her supervisor to think she is incompetent and that her focus is placed on how she is perceived by her supervisor as opposed to how to repair ruptures in-session with her client. Susan decides to present these observations to her client and asks for her client's impression on how the therapeutic relationship has felt.

In this vignette, there are three major points. First, supervisors must recognize that supervisees' therapeutic alliance does not necessarily happen when both therapists and clients are "feeling good" about each other. There are processes that are leading up to therapeutic alliance that, at times, feels extremely broken. However, with careful examination and reflective processes, it is possible for supervisees to recognize that even in emotionally volatile situations good therapists unconsciously mirror their clients' emotionality. Susan's tendency to shut down when her client was shutting down in therapy is an example of this. Second, a gentle but firm reminder to supervisees that when they are in therapeutic situations, as hard as it may be, having full attention on their clients is absolutely necessary. Susan's focus shifting away from her client and onto her wanting to appear competent in her supervisor's eyes changed her therapeutic interactions. As her supervisor noticed, just as Susan's client felt that Susan was concentrating on something other than her, she indeed "acted out" more. Because her client was not capable or willing to communicate this to Susan— that she wanted Susan's full attention—she would behave in a way that would demand Susan to return focus on her. Third, none of these observations can be reported back to supervisors by their supervisees. Without relying on factual recordings of therapy sessions or live supervision, supervisees would not be able to capture the intricate and complex dynamics that emerge in therapy with their clients. It is crucial for supervisors to observe exact moments when dynamics change between supervisees and their clients in therapy and use these moments to elicit self-reflections from supervisees. Supervisees simply and verbally reporting back their experiences with their clients would only be filtered by their conscious frameworks, which are often tempered by elements that would impact their impressions.

Managing Countertransference

Strupp (1980) noted that among the "major decrements to the foundation of a good working alliance are . . . the therapist's personal reactions" (p. 953). One of the more challenging tasks for novice therapists is to stay present with their clients regardless of what feelings or reactions their clients or situations elicit. In fact, this can be true of even the best trained and intentioned therapists (Ackerman & Hilsenroth, 2001). This, then, is an important training focus for supervision.

It is useful to consider four supervisory targets in helping supervisees recognize and manage countertransference (see, e.g., Hayes et al., 1998; Ladany, Friedlander, & Nelson, 2005).

1. *Identifying what triggered the reactions*: These usually concern something (a) about the session content, (b) about the characteristics of the client, or

(c) about particular processes that are occurring in the therapy (Hayes & Gelso, 2001).

2. *Identifying origins of the supervisee's reactions*: This speaks to the source of the supervisees' reactions, which could include, for example, their family history, needs and values, or multicultural issues (Hayes et al., 1998; Ligiero & Gelso, 2002).

3. *Identifying the markers of countertransference*: These concern the supervisee's reactions and how those reactions are then affecting objectivity. The supervisee may readily recognize when this is occurring and bring it to the supervisor (e.g., "I find myself so bored with this client that I have difficulty concentrating when he talks"). Or, in other cases, the supervisor might notice some behavior (e.g., the supervisee changes the subject whenever a particular topic comes up) that the supervisee has not noticed.

4. *Management*: This is the action-oriented portion of the supervision: what will the supervisee do to minimize the intrusion of the countertransference in his or her work?

It is in working with countertransference that the supervisor is most vulnerable to the ethical risk of veering into the role of the supervisee's therapist (Goodyear & Rodolfa, 2012). Processing countertransference needs to remain anchored in the supervisee's work with the specific client; there usually is scant reason to do more in supervision with the origins of countertransference (see earlier discussion) than to perhaps acknowledge them.

Some of the supervisor's questions to the supervisee might include:

1. What distracts you from truly seeing the client's challenges, strengths, and therapeutic needs?

2. What specific support do you need from me (the supervisor) to focus on building a strong alliance with your client? Are there factors about our own supervisor–supervisee relationship that affect how you are or are not able to form an alliance with your client?

3. If we were to recognize that the techniques we choose are based on the strength of alliance we have with our clients, what specific techniques would you choose for your client at this point in your therapeutic care and why?

Countertransference affects how the therapist reacts affectively or interpersonally to the client, and, as Gelso and Mohr (2001) observe, "if countertransference is not understood by the therapist or managed in one way or another, it is likely to impede the formation of working alliance and erode an existing alliance" (p. 57). Helping supervisees learn to identify and manage countertransference, therefore, should be a core focus of any supervision efforts to establish and maintain supervisees' alliances with their clients.

Developing Self-Care Competencies

Supervisees' capacity to build and maintain alliances relies on their having sufficient levels of self-awareness and empathy, "entering the private, perceptual world of the other" (Norcross & Hill, 2004, p. 20). Helping them develop those attributes is an important focus of supervision. But self-awareness and empathic attunement can be affected by a therapist's life circumstances and personal stress. Therefore, an important—but too-often overlooked—goal for supervisors is helping supervisees learn and commit to self-care strategies that will become life-long habits. In fact, Barnett, Johnston, and Hillard (2005) went so far as to assert that this is an ethical imperative.

In the worst cases, failure to be effective in self-care can lead to the emotional exhaustion and sense of depersonalization that are hallmarks of burnout (Maslach & Jackson, 1981). But whereas burnout is a real risk for a subset of psychotherapists, the more acute experience of distress is much more pervasive. Guy, Poelstra, and Stark (1989) found that three-fourths of their sample of psychologists acknowledged having experienced distress during the past 3 years, and more than a third of those indicated that this had negatively affected the quality of their care to clients. One specific effect is on clinical decision-making which, in turn, relates to quality of client care (Norcross, 2000) and how it would negatively affect both the supervisory and the therapist–client alliance.

Smith and Moss (2009) posited that therapists who neglect self-care should be vigilant for signs of exhaustion, depression, and vicarious traumatization. If the habits of self-care are to be life-long, they should begin in graduate school. Yet Doran (2014), speaking as then-chair of the American Psychological Association of Graduate Students, noted how graduate students' fear of being behind on all that they are responsible for (i.e., coursework, clinical training, teaching, and writing for publications and dissertation) is a substantial detriment to self-care. Even when admonished to engage in self-care, many students hear this as simply another demand (though regrettably, it is the demand for which their faculty and supervisors may be least likely to hold them accountable).

Supervisors might employ self-care guidelines such as those of Ungar, Mackey, Guest, and Bernard (2000). They could assist and remind supervisees of the importance of self-care by having conversations with them that begin with the following questions:

1. What do you imagine would be the consequences to you clients of not attending to your own self-care? Let's talk about the ramifications of emotional, relational, and ethical impacts of that.
2. Imagine yourself as one of your clients. What would you tell yourself if you do not get enough sleep, eat well, and take some time to enjoy life, family, and friends?
3. If it is that you are not able to practice what you preach to your clients about self-care, how would you like to change that? What support and resources are needed for you to make that change?

Summary

In writing this chapter, we were mindful of Muran et al.'s (2011) observation that "every intervention has relational meaning" (p. 321). This is true in supervision as well. Every intervention we discussed here has relational implications with the supervisee, and, given the interlocking nature of supervision and therapy, those relational phenomena have some likelihood of being transmitted to the supervisee's work with clients. Perhaps this is another way of asserting that almost all that supervisors do has some implication for supervisees' developing abilities to develop and manage alliances.

There are only a few other relationships as impactful and transformative as that of supervisors and supervised during graduate school—if done right. They frame and provide the contextual foundation necessary for supervisees to begin forming therapeutic alliances with their own clients. When we venture into new types of relationships we rely on previous relationships to understand and create the new relationships' rules while negotiating reactions to discomfort to newness or differences, and the same process happens when supervisees begin working with their clients to form alliances. Although there are core and critical elements that foster alliance, there is no one simple formula that would work for all relationships. What we have shared in this chapter, hopefully, are a few of core concepts and matters that influence the outcome of the process of alliance building.

References

Ackerman, S. J., & Hilsenroth, M. J. (2001). A review of therapist characteristics and techniques negatively impacting the therapeutic alliance. *Psychotherapy: Theory, Research, Practice, Training, 38*(2), 171–185.

Alegria, M., Canino, G., Shrout, P. E., Woo. M., Duan. N., Vila. D., Torres, M., Chen, C. N., & Meng, X. L. (2008). Prevalence of mental illness in immigrant and non-immingrant U.S. Latino groups. *American Journal of Psychiatry*, *165*(3), 359–369.

American Psychological Association (APA). (2015). Guidelines for clinical supervision in health service psychology. *American Psychologist*, *70*, 33–46.

Amerikaner, M., & Rose, T. (2012). Direct observation of psychology supervisees' clinical work: A snapshot of current practice. *The Clinical Supervisor*, *31*(1), 61–80.

Anderson, T., Crowley, M. E. J., Himawan, L., Holmberg, J. K., & Uhlin, B. D. (2016). Therapist facilitative interpersonal skills and training status: A randomized clinical trial on alliance and outcome. *Psychotherapy Research*, *26*(5), 511–529.

Anderson, T., McClintock, A. S., Himawan, L., Song, X., & Patterson, C. L. (2016). A prospective study of therapist facilitative interpersonal skills as a predictor of treatment outcome. *Journal of Consulting and Clinical Psychology*, *84*(1), 57–66.

Baldwin, S. A., Wampold, B. E., & Imel, Z. E. (2007). Untangling the alliance–outcome correlation: Exploring the relative importance of therapist and patient variability in the alliance. *Journal of Consulting and Clinical Psychology*, *75*, 842–852. doi:10.1037/0022-006X.75.6.842

Bambling, M., King, R., Raue, P., Schweitzer, R., & Lambert, W. (2006). Clinical supervision: Its influence on client-rated working alliance and client symptom reduction in the brief treatment of major depression. *Psychotherapy Research*, *16*(03), 317–331.

Barlow, D. H. (2014). *Clinical handbook of psychological disorders: A step-by-step treatment manual* (5th ed.). New York: Guilford Press.

Barnett, J. E., Johnston, L. C., & Hillard, D. (2006). Psychotherapist wellness as an ethical imperative. In L. VandeCreek& J. B. Allen (Eds.), *Innovations in Clinical Practice: Focus on Health and Wellness* (pp. 257–271). Professional Resources Press, Sarasota, FL.

Bernard, J. M., & Goodyear, R. K. (2019). *Fundamentals of clinical supervision*. (6th edition). Boston: Merrill.

Borders, L. D., Cashwell, C. S., & Rotter, J. C. (1995). Supervision of counselor licensure applicants: A comparative study. *Counselor Education and Supervision*, *35*(1), 54–69.

Bordin, E. S. (1979). The generalizability of the psychoanalytic concept of the working alliance. *Psychotherapy: Theory, research & practice*, *16*(3), 252–260.

Boswell, J. F., Kraus, D. R., Miller, S. D., & Lambert, M. J. (2015). Implementing routine outcome monitoring in clinical practice: Benefits, challenges, and solutions. *Psychotherapy Research*, *25*(1), 6–19.

Castonguay, L. G., Goldfried, M. R., Wiser, S., Raue, P. J., & Hayes, A. M. (1996). Predicting the effect of cognitive therapy for depression: A study of unique and common factors. *Journal of Consulting and Clinical Psychology*, *64*(3), 497–504.

Chow, D. L., Miller, S. D., Seidel, J. A., Kane, R. T., Thornton, J. A., & Andrews, W. P. (2015). The role of deliberate practice in the development of highly effective psychotherapists. *Psychotherapy*, *52*(3), 337–345.

Croucher, S. M., Bruno, A., McGrath, P., Adams, C., McGahan, C., Suits, A., & Huckins, A. (2012). Conflict styles and high–low context cultures: A cross-cultural extension. *Communication Research Reports*, *29*(1), 64–73.

Doran, J. M. (2014). The unspoken truth about self-care. *GradPsych*, *12*(2), 48.

Ellis, M. V., Berger, L., Hanus, A. E., Ayala, E. E., Swords, B. A., & Siembor, M. (2014). Inadequate and harmful clinical supervision: Testing a revised framework and assessing occurrence. *The Counseling Psychologist*, *42*(4), 434–472.

Ermold, J., Lefkowitz, C., & Santanello, A. (n.d.). Practical for your practice: Delivering an effective treatment rationale. Uniformed Services University, Department of Deployment Psychology. Video, available online at https://vimeo.com/188832364

Ericsson, K. A., Krampe, R. T., & Tesch-Römer, C. (1993). The role of deliberate practice in the acquisition of expert performance. *Psychological Review, 100*(3), 363–406.

Eubanks-Carter, C., Muran, J. C., & Safran, J. D. (2015). Alliance-focused training. *Psychotherapy, 52*(2), 169–173.

Flückiger, C., Del Re, A. C., Wampold, B. E., & Horvath, A. O. (2018). The alliance in adult psychotherapy: A meta-analytic synthesis. *Psychotherapy, 55*(4), 316–340.

Frank, J. D., & Frank, J. B. (1993). *Persuasion and healing: A comparative study of psychotherapy.* Baltimore, MD: Johns Hopkins University Press.

Gallo, J. J., Marino, S., Ford, D., & Anthony, J. C. (1995). Filters on the pathway to mental health care, II. Sociodemographic factors. *Psychological Medicine, 25*(6), 1149–1160.

Geller, J. D., Farber, B. A., & Schaffer, C. E. (2010). Representations of the supervisory dialogue and the development of psychotherapists. *Psychotherapy: Theory, Research, Practice, Training, 47*(2), 211–220.

Gelso, C. (2014). A tripartite model of the therapeutic relationship: Theory, research, and practice. *Psychotherapy Research, 24*(2), 117–131.

Gelso, C. J., & Mohr, J. J. (2001). The working alliance and the transference/countertransference relationship: Their manifestation with racial/ethnic and sexual orientation minority clients and therapists. *Applied and Preventive Psychology, 10*(1), 51–68.

Gladwell, M. (2008). *Outliers: The story of success.* New York: Little, Brown.

Goldberg, S. B., Babins-Wagner, R., Rousmaniere, T., Berzins, S., Hoyt, W. T., Whipple, J. L., . . . Wampold, B. E. (2016). Creating a climate for therapist improvement: A case study of an agency focused on outcomes and deliberate practice. *Psychotherapy, 53*(3), 367–375.

Goldberg, S. B., Rousmaniere, T., Miller, S. D., Whipple, J., Nielsen, S. L., Hoyt, W. T., & Wampold, B. E. (2016). Do psychotherapists improve with time and experience? A longitudinal analysis of outcomes in a clinical setting. *Journal of Counseling Psychology, 63*(1), 1–11.

Goodyear, R. K. (Producer). (1982) . Psychotherapy supervision by major theorists. Manhattan: Kansas State University.

Goodyear, R. K. (2014). Supervision as pedagogy: Attending to its essential instructional and learning processes. *The Clinical Supervisor, 33*(1), 82–99.

Goodyear, R. K., & Rodolfa, E. (2012). Negotiating the complex ethical terrain of clinical supervision. In S. Knapp (Ed.), *Handbook on ethics in psychology* (pp. 261–276). Washington, DC: American Psychological Association.

Gudykunst, W. B., & Nishida, T. (1986). Attributional confidence in low and high-context cultures. *Human Communication Research, 12,* 525–549.

Guest, P. D., & Beutler, L. E. (1988). Impact of psychotherapy supervision on therapist orientation and values. *Journal of Consulting and Clinical Psychology, 56*(5), 653–658.

Guy, J. D., Poelstra, P. L., & Stark, M. J. (1989). Professional distress and therapeutic effectiveness: National survey of psychologists practicing psychotherapy. *Professional Psychology: Research and Practice, 20*(1), 48–50.

Haggerty, G., & Hilsenroth, M. J. (2011). The use of video in psychotherapy supervision. *British Journal of Psychotherapy, 27*(2), 193–210.

Hayes, J. A., & Gelso, C. J. (2001). Clinical implications of research on countertransference: Science informing practice. *Journal of Clinical Psychology, 57*(8), 1041–1051.

Hayes, J. A., McCracken, J. E., McClanahan, M. K., Hill, C. E., Harp, J. S., & Carozzoni, P. (1998). Therapist perspectives on countertransference: Qualitative data in search of a theory. *Journal of Counseling Psychology, 45*(4), 468–482.

Henry, W. P., Strupp, H. H., Butler, S. F., Schacht, T. E., & Binder, J. L. (1993). Effects of training in time-limited dynamic psychotherapy: Changes in therapist behavior. *Journal of Consulting and Clinical Psychology, 61*(3), 434–440.

Hersoug, A. G., Monsen, J. T., Havik, O. E., & Høglend, P. (2002). Quality of early working alliance in psychotherapy: Diagnoses, relationship and intrapsychic variables as predictors. *Psychotherapy and Psychosomatics, 71*(1), 18–27.

Hill, C. E. (2014). *Helping skills: Facilitating exploration, insight, and action.* Washington, DC: American Psychological Association.

Hill, C. E., Gelso, C. J., Chui, H., Spangler, P. T., Hummel, A., Huang, T., . . . Gupta, S. (2014). To be or not to be immediate with clients: The use and perceived effects of immediacy in psychodynamic/interpersonal psychotherapy. *Psychotherapy Research, 24*(3), 299–315.

Hill, C. E., & Knox, S. (2009). Processing the therapeutic relationship. *Psychotherapy Research, 19*(1), 13–29.

Howard, K. I., Moras, K., Brill, P. L., Martinovich, Z., & Lutz, W. (1996). Efficacy, effectiveness, and patient progress. *American Psychologist, 51*, 1059–1064.

Kagan, N. I., & Kagan, H. (1990). IPR-A validated model for the 1990s and beyond. *The Counseling Psychologist, 18*(3), 436–440.

Kiesler, D. J. (1988). *Therapeutic metacommunication.* Palo Alto, CA: Consulting Psychologist Press.

Knox, S. (2015). Disclosure—and lack thereof—in individual supervision. *The Clinical Supervisor, 34*(2), 151–163.

Ladany, N., Friedlander, M. L., & Nelson, M. L. (2005). *Critical events in psychotherapy supervision: An interpersonal approach.* Washington, DC: American Psychological Association.

Lambert, M. J. (2015). Progress feedback and the OQ-system: The past and the future. *Psychotherapy, 52*(4), 381–390.

Ligiero, D. P, & Gelso, C. J. (2002). Countertransference, attachment, and the working alliance: The therapist's contribution. *Psychotherapy Theory Research and Practice, 39*(1), 3–11.

Maslach, C., & Jackson, S. E. (1981). The measurement of experienced burnout. *Journal of Organizational Behavior, 2*(2), 99–113.

Miller, S. D., Duncan, B. L., Sorrell, R., & Brown, G. S. (2005). The Partners for Change Outcome Management System. *Journal of Clinical Psychology: In-Session, 61*, 199–208.

Miller, S. D., Hubble, M. A., & Chow, D. (2017). Professional development: From oxymoron to reality. In T. Rousmaniere, R. Goodyear, S. Miller, & B. Wampold (Eds.), *The cycle of excellence: Using deliberate practice to improve supervision and training* (pp. 23–49). New York: Wiley.

Muran, J. C., Safran, J. D., & Eubanks-Carter, C. (2011). Developing therapist abilities to negotiate alliance ruptures. In J. J. Muran & J. P. Barber (Eds.), *The therapeutic alliance: An evidence-based guide to practice* (pp. 320–340). New York: Guilford Press.

Muslin, H. L., Thurnblad, R. J., & Meschel, G. (1981). The fate of the clinical interview: An observational study. *American Journal of Psychiatry, 138,* 822–825.

Norcross, J. C. (2000). Psychotherapist self-care: Practitioner-tested, research-informed strategies. *Professional Psychology Research and Practice, 31*(6), 710–713.

Norcross, J. C., & Hill, C. E. (2004). Empirically supported therapy relationships. *The Clinical Psychologist, 57*(3), 19–24.

Owen, J., & Hilsenroth, M. J. (2014). Treatment adherence: The importance of therapist flexibility in relation to therapy outcomes. *Journal of Counseling Psychology, 61*(2), 280–288.

Park, Y. S., & Kim, B. S. K. (2008). Asian and European American cultural values and communication styles among Asian Americans and European American college students. *Cultural Diversity and Ethnic Minority Psychology, 14*(1), 47–56.

Patton, M. J., & Kivlighan Jr., D. M. (1997). Relevance of the supervisory alliance to the counseling alliance and to treatment adherence in counselor training. *Journal of Counseling Psychology, 44*(1), 108–115.

Price, T. G., Roberts, C. E., Fatollahi, J. J., & Gandhi, B. S. (2016). Teaching professionalism and countertransference to psychiatric residents. *Psychiatric Annals, 46*(5), 298–302.

Raven, B. H. (2008). The bases of power and the power/interaction model of interpersonal influence. *Analyses of Social Issues and Public Policy, 8*(1), 1–22.

Shafran, N., Kivlighan, D. M., Gelso, C. J., Bhatia, A., & Hill, C. E. (2017). Therapist immediacy: The association with working alliance, real relationship, session quality, and time in psychotherapy. *Psychotherapy Research, 27*(6), 737-748.

Sharf, J., Primavera, L. H., & Diener, M. J. (2010). Dropout and therapeutic alliance: A meta-analysis of adult individual psychotherapy. *Psychotherapy: Theory, Research, Practice, Training, 47*(4), 637–645.

Smith, P. L., & Moss, S. B. (2009). Psychologist impairment: What is it, how can it be prevented, and what can be done to address it? *Clinical Psychology Science and Practice, 16*(1), 1–15.

Stoltenberg, C. D., Bailey, K. C., Cruzan, C. B., Hart, J. T., & Ukuku, U. (2014). The integrative developmental model of supervision. In C. E. Watkins, Jr. & D. Milne (Eds.), *Wiley international handbook of clinical supervision* (pp. 576–597). Chichester, UK: John Wiley & Sons.

Strupp, H. H. (1980). Success and failure in time-limited psychotherapy further evidence (Comparison 4). *Archives of General Psychiatry, 37,* 947–954.

Sue, S., & Zane, N. (2009). The role of culture and cultural techniques in psychotherapy: A critique and reformulation. *Asian American Journal of Psychology, S*(1), 3–14.

Swift, J. K., Callahan, J. L., Rousmaniere, T. G., Whipple, J. L., Dexter, K., & Wrape, E. R. (2015). Using client outcome monitoring as a tool for supervision. *Psychotherapy, 52,* 180–184.

Ungar, M., Mackey, L., Guest, M., & Bernard, C. (2000). Logotherapeutic guidelines for therapists' self-care. *International Forum for Logotherapy, 23*(2), 89–94.

Wampold, B. E. (2017). What should we practice? A contextual model for how psychotherapy works. In T. Rousmaniere, R. K. Goodyear, S. D. Miller, & B. E. Wampold (Eds.), *The cycle of excellence* (pp. 49–65). Hoboken, NJ: John Wiley & Sons.

Wampold, B. E., & Imel, Z. E. (2015). *The great psychotherapy debate: The evidence for what makes psychotherapy work.* New York, NY: Routledge.

Watzlawick, P., Beavin, J. H., & Jackson, D. D. (1967). *Pragmatics of human communication: A study of interactional patterns, pathologies, and paradoxes.* New York: Norton.

White, M. B., & Russell, C. S. (1997). Examining the multifaceted notion of isomorphism in marriage and family therapy supervision: A quest for conceptual clarity. *Journal of Marital and Family Therapy, 23*(3), 315–333.

Wynne, M. E., Susman, M., Ries, S., Birringer, J., & Katz, L. (1994). A method for assessing therapists' recall of in-session events. *Journal of Counseling Psychology, 41*(1), 53–57.

Yourman, D. B., & Farber, B. A. (1996). Nondisclosure and distortion in psychotherapy supervision. *Psychotherapy: Theory, Research, Practice, Training, 33*(4), 567–575.

10

Integration and Discussion

Jairo N. Fuertes

I set out to produce a book that could answer a thoughtful student's question: "How do I go about creating a working alliance with a client?" As noted in the introduction, while I was very familiar with the research on the working alliance, had conducted a few studies on the topic, and had taught and trained many students about the importance of the working alliance, I really did not know how to answer such a direct and practical question. Despite having had excellent graduate-level education and clinical experience that included having worked successfully with many clients, I came to realize that no one had ever taught me how to actually go about establishing the working alliance with a client. In thinking about the way to address this question, it became evident that this would require a book-length treatise as a response, and the contributions of other colleagues who have been thinking and writing about this topic for some time. I hope that, despite the long response, we have been successful in answering this question. In this chapter, I will provide an integration and discussion of the main points, as I see them, from each of the previous chapters.

So, what do the authors say about what is needed to create a working alliance? It is clear that a working alliance does not just happen: it has to be cultivated and maintained, at times even repaired. Simply putting together a well-meaning therapist and a motivated client in a counseling room does not guarantee that a working alliance will develop between the two. While the working alliance is a collaborative effort and product, it is the therapist's primary job to foster its development, along with the contributions and collaboration of the client. Finding a shared focus and purpose to the work is at the heart of what constitutes the working alliance, and this is exactly what the therapist must set to accomplish from the earliest moments in treatment. We can assume that the client has some level of motivation or interest to work on a problem, otherwise why would the client be in the counselor's office? But as noted by Bedi and Hayes, the client is often ambivalent about their situation, the client is usually in some level of emotional discomfort, and a readiness to focus or a clear sense of purpose or direction may not be readily available to the client. The therapist must harness focus and purpose, with the client, in order to make the working alliance a possibility.

Why is training in working alliance skills so important? Several authors note the outcome research, which has shown that therapy is remarkably effective and that the working alliance is a consistent predictor of good things being achieved in therapy. However, missteps and misunderstandings (or, as Gardner et al. in Chapter 8 refer to them, "misattunements") can easily lead to a relatively negative experience for both people, with the client possibly bearing the brunt of an unfruitful exchange. While this is rare, it happens. In fact, we know that therapy does not always go well. While therapy is very helpful to many people, there is premature termination in therapy, sometimes after just one session, and, in rare cases, a small percentage of clients make absolutely no gains from treatment or even get worse while being in treatment (Lambert, 2013). I will not suggest that this is due solely to a weak working alliance; it is difficult to determine why a small percentage of clients do not benefit from therapy. What we do know is that therapy is most effective when a working alliance develops very early in therapy, although it waxes and wanes in strength throughout treatment (Lambert, 2013). Even in therapies where a heavy emphasis is placed on techniques and procedures, keeping a focus on the working alliance is conducive to good outcomes. Training in working alliance skills can help students, new professionals, and even seasoned clinicians improve their ability to help an array of clients. This training need not take away from what therapists already do successfully with their clients; instead, it can help them become more effective in facilitating/producing clinically significant change.

The discussion here is organized in terms of factors or variables that refer primarily (though not exclusively) to either the therapist, the client, or their interactions.

The Therapist

Hatcher and Barends (2006) noted that the alliance is the result of multiple components acting together, not an isolated component. Relatedly, in Chapter 3, Anderson and Perlman noted that working alliance competence can be achieved not by focusing on learning treatment manuals or memorizing specific protocols based on specific therapies, but by attending to crucial facilitative and interpersonal skills. These authors also note something important to reiterate here: that competence as a therapist involves a life-long learning process, so please allow yourself to learn—you can still be very helpful to clients without being the perfect or near-perfect therapist—and try to enjoy the long but satisfying journey of learning and improving as a clinician.

A perusal of the chapters points to the important and central role of therapist skills, knowledge, and attitudes in fostering the working alliance. The skills, knowledge, and attitudes presented in the chapters are not a new—they are skills that are already known to and used by counselors—but they can be used deliberately to create and fortify the working alliance. These three therapist factors serve to set the stage for the work of counseling and help to prepare, activate, and engage the client, who is also a crucial player in the alliance. A prominent theme is the role of the therapist in creating the conditions for the working alliance to emerge through a variety of interventions that are largely client-centered or Rogerian (i.e., warmth, empathy, unconditional positive regard for the client). Perez et al., in Chapter 2, refer to these qualities as "trust potentiating" for the client, and the emotional experience of trust between a client and a therapist is foundational to therapy. Some level of trust has to be in place in order for goals and tasks to become possible. As Hatcher and Barends (2006) suggest, the working alliance is built from the ground up, one interaction at a time, through the use of skills, knowledge, and attitudes that are conveyed to the client.

In terms of skills, therapist-offered empathy stands out as a skill frequently referenced by several authors as essential to alliance development. Empathy is discussed as a foundational skill that facilitates connecting with, understanding, and planning treatment with the client. Tryon, in Chapter 4, discusses how empathy makes the selection of meaningful and attainable goals possible, as well as the selection of tasks needed to achieve them. Another skill that is referenced, despite being generally considered an advanced skill (Hill, 2014), is therapist immediacy. Several authors allude to immediacy as a mechanism for helping therapists check in with their clients on how they feel about the direction of therapy and to obtain feedback and input from their clients. While questions and probes are also identified as valuable, there seems to be an interpersonal quality to immediacy that conveys the sense of clients and therapists being together in a working relationship. Another set of skills that is mentioned in several chapters is therapists' use of nonverbal behaviors that convey attention, warmth, and interest in the client. Attention to clients' nonverbal behaviors can also offer valuable cues about what the client may be experiencing or feeling in the session.

Several authors make reference to the use of facilitative interpersonal skills (FIS), and these skills are featured prominently in Chapter 3. These "skills" or capacities represent pan-theoretical pragmatic methods that can be cultivated and used to enhance the working alliance. The work of Anderson and his collaborators has generated empirical support for the use of FIS to improve outcomes and working alliances. These skills include abilities in emotional expression, in persuasion, and in generating positive expectations, and they appear to be most valuable during challenging moments in therapy. FIS are interesting in their novelty in that they represent more than helping skills: they are therapist relational capacities that can be cultivated to improve the effectiveness of therapy via interpersonal processes. Anderson and Perlman (Chapter 3) also discuss the role of therapist responsiveness—the ability to detect and modify in-session processes based on subtle, interpersonal shifts in the client's expression and communication. Therapist responsiveness and the use of FIS is of particular importance during challenging, emotionally charged incidents during therapy, known as "critical relational markers." These authors indicate that FIS can be fostered through deliberate practice, and they mention in their chapter the development of a very promising FIS training program, Facilitative Interpersonal Relationship Skills Training (FIRST), that encompasses four separate modules designed sequentially to build on successively more complex skills.

Several authors mention therapists conveying an attitude that communicates respect to the client. As a clinician, it seems hard to overemphasize this last point. The client is the person who knows the client best and, in my opinion, is the most important person in the working alliance. Conveying respect to the client empowers the client as well as the therapist, and, by empowering the client, respect facilitates the process of finding focus, direction, and purpose to the work. Therapist humility is also discussed as an attitude that conveys respect as well as an interest in learning and working together collaboratively with the client. Respect and humility feature prominently as essential attitudes to developing a working alliance when Duan (Chapter 7) and Goodyear and Sera (Chapter 9) discuss establishing the working alliance with clients (and supervisees working with clients) from historically oppressed and marginalized populations.

Therapists' attitudes and knowledge also include self-awareness and a deep self-understanding; these are discussed by several authors as important in today's complex, international, and multicultural society. The old adage "Therapist know thyself" has never rung more true. Duan (Chapter 7) and Gerald et al. (Chapter 8) note the value of mindfulness in yielding self-understanding of intrapsychic and interpersonal dynamics, including alliance ruptures and managing client transference and countertransference. Egan's (2010) idea of creating a "just society" with clients, one based on mutual respect, fairness, and collaboration, is also referenced in two different chapters—the spirit of justice is conveyed in how the therapist approaches the client, but it is also informed by therapists' knowledge and understanding of the role of inequity, poverty, oppression, and marginalization in society. Deliberate practice (Rousmaniere, 2016) is noted by several authors as a way of targeting the needed skills and behaviors that facilitate working alliance competence. Goodyear and Sera (Chapter 9) note how supervisors can facilitate the deliberate development of alliance skills. For example, supervisors can target specific therapist behaviors to practice with their supervisees in supervision, they can provide practice assignments between supervision sessions, they can provide feedback to supervisees based on videotaped counseling, and they can model optimal behaviors in developing an alliance in supervision that supervisees can carry over and use in counseling.

The Client

It is evident from reading the chapters that the client is as important, if not more important than the therapist to the development and sustainment of the working alliance in treatment. Without the client's efforts and collaboration, even the best of therapists are doomed to fail in that their interventions and efforts will have little to no effect on outcome. Several authors remind us that clients bring with them unique personal experiences, perspectives, and values, and that they form subjective impressions of the therapist (and therapy) which are influenced by culture and ethnoracial status. These client factors need to be assessed, understood, and included in the development of the working alliance. Bedi and Hayes (Chapter 6) highlight findings from research that show that clients form their own views of the working alliance, and while these views are like those of their therapists, their views are also distinct from their therapists'. Bedi and Hayes go on to suggest that clients' views need to be accounted for and integrated into the treatment. After all, how can consensus and collaboration take hold in a relationship if the agenda for the work in such a relationship has been dictated by only one of the participants? In order to achieve "agreement" about the goals and tasks of treatment, both client and therapist need to have presented their ideas and collaboratively worked on the focus and direction of therapy. Also, it seems clear that while every therapist offers a form of treatment (e.g., some variation of cognitive-behavior therapy or of short-term psychodynamic therapy), it is the client who has to do much of the work of behavior change. And it is the client who can reap the benefits from his or her efforts, or inversely, it's the client who has to contend with unexpected results, such as realizing that a marriage is not salvageable, or realizing that he or she really does not want to study pre-med in college despite parents' wishes. Fuertes & Williams (2017) compared the work of the client in therapy to that of the person who seeks physical fitness in a gym. The person can get instruction, support, and motivation from a personal trainer, but, ultimately, they have to go through the rigors of physical training, the workouts, the sore muscles, to gain physical fitness. Similarly, in therapy, the client has to do the workout. In counseling, the exercises are reflection, honest communication, collaboration with the therapist and other people, and planning and engaging in behavior change. The client does most of the work, with the support and assistance of the therapist and, ultimately, has to contend with the results.

Several authors also point to the results of meta-analyses that have examined the effects of the working alliance on outcome, which include the finding that clients' ratings of the working alliance are strongly associated with outcome. If a client has been able to establish a trusting and productive relationship with a therapist, one in which some goals have been attained, then ratings of outcome will be high. However, as Bedi and Hayes (Chapter 6) point out, what is deemed as trusting and productive (and helpful) will vary from client to client. Furthermore, Duan (Chapter 7) notes that each client (and each therapist, for that matter) is a complex personality made up of multiple self-identities, and these identities (e.g., based on race or sexual orientation or socioeconomic status) may need to be recognized and attended to in the working alliance and in therapy. The point to be highlighted here is that there is no such thing as a nominal client; no therapy dyad and no therapy session is ever replicated—each is different and unique. Each working alliance is unique to the particular dyad at work and is shaped and characterized by the identities seeking expression in the relationship at any given point. This makes the job of treatment interesting and challenging—the therapist must always be "on" for the client, flexible, adaptive, and receptive to the needs that the client is expressing or needs to express in therapy. Tryon (Chapter 4) and Fuertes et al. (Chapter 5) discuss how clients' values and beliefs and their hopes and ideas about the future need to be centrally incorporated into the treatment plan. While therapists can also have input as part of the collaborative process, the client's input is of utmost importance. Going back to the analogy of the physical gym, clients are most likely to do the workout and sustain the hard work of behavior change if the goals and tasks that they have set for themselves have intrinsic worth and value. Having established open lines of communication, client feedback will be essential if goals or tasks need to be modified and/or changed, and client input is crucial in properly assessing/monitoring progress in treatment. In sum, as noted by Fuertes et al. in Chapter 5, clients have to experience having control and say in the direction of therapy: they should experience therapy as happening because of them, instead of happening "to them."

Therapist–Client Interactions

While therapist and client factors are important variables that have to be considered with respect to the development of the working alliance, their interactions—that is, what transpires between therapist and client—goes to the heart of the working alliance. The goal in the alliance is to foster the sense of being an "ally" to the client, of being for him or her, of being thoroughly aligned for the client's well-being. A few points from the chapters are worth noting: for example, several authors note the importance of very early impressions to the formation of the working alliance—particularly early impressions by the client. The working alliance begins from the very first contact and sets in motion a process of relating that can yield that sense of being allies—or not, which would be detrimental to the work. So, from the very first contact, the therapist has to convey a genuine interest in understanding and connecting with the client and in conveying an abiding disposition to help. Bedi and Hayes (Chapter 6) note that part of the process in the first session might be to assess how the client is experiencing the session and what their perceptions are of the therapist, the office, etc. Making this verbal, and therefore something that can be processed, can help allay inhibitions or offset any negative first impressions. Given the evidence that the client might have differing perceptions of the session/therapy experience, a conscious effort to align perceptions early in therapy, in a way that fosters collaboration, is important (e.g., by inviting and/or allowing the client to express how he or she feels in the room after a few minutes with the therapist; or perhaps the therapist conveys a desire to be on the same page with the client and wanting the work to be collaborative in nature; these might be good first steps at practicing genuine communication and in helping the client feel more comfortable with sharing his or her feelings). If the client begins to feel more comfortable communicating feelings and thoughts, this can be invaluable in helping to formulate and calibrate goals and tasks for therapy. Fuertes et al. (Chapter 5) note that while the motivation that a client brings on his or her own to therapy is important, motivation that develops in collaboration with the therapist may be as important in following through with the actual tasks and goals of therapy.

Tryon (Chapter 4) highlights the importance of the therapist and client working together to set attainable goals and that working together may be important in the process of making seemingly unattainable goals more attainable for the client. This "working together" implies a back-and-forth process of sharing and negotiating, collaboratively monitoring and re-evaluating the progress made, and discussing the viability of goals and tasks that have been implemented. At a strategic level, Fuertes et al. (Chapter 5) note the use of "us and "we" pronouns to highlight the shared mission of the work even in situations and therapies where goals or tasks have not been explicitly set. Another important aspect of therapist–client interactions involves therapists' abilities to identify, process, and solve ruptures in the working alliance. Gardner et al. (Chapter 8) present examples of both withdrawal and confrontation ruptures, behaviors that can challenge the work and the progress in treatment. They also provide corresponding examples of interventions that can help heal these ruptures through the use immediate (i.e., an immediate intervention) or expressive (i.e., a more depth-oriented process of exploration) repair strategies.

The "working" part of the working alliance certainly alludes to activity, or action. Fuertes et al. (Chapter 5) refer to action as a collaborative effort as well, jointly planned and monitored. Clients who have been able to experience an alliance in the work will feel that they have the support and encouragement of their therapist. Instead of feeling like they are taking on the process of change on their own, they have the sense that they are in a joint venture together with their therapist. This is important as well with the process of termination. While therapy comes to an end at some point, the client who has experienced a collaborative alliance with his or her therapist is in a better position to establish collaborations with others outside of the therapy. In other words, the working alliance helps patients beyond the parameters of therapy, that is, beyond termination. Tryon (Chapter 4) also points out that the process of working as allies helps the client attain goals, but it does not mean that perfect goal attainment is needed for success. Achieving some goals but not others, or achieving some aspects or parts of a goal, may be sufficient to help the client move forward. The experience of having some success with behavior change can also motivate the client to pursue other goals, either in another future therapy experience or outside of therapy, with the support of family or other community resources. In other words, beyond goal attainment and task completion, the working alliance can help clients gain a sense of momentum and direction in a positive direction and enhance their capacity to collaborate with others outside of therapy.

Some authors also note that there may be different types of working alliances. For the purpose of the book, I purposely delimited the scope of inquiry by having the authors focus on the working alliance as proposed by Bordin (1979; i.e., in terms of goals, tasks, bond). But in the Introduction, we mention other measures of the alliance, and we also note the results of factor analyses examining various measures, which show that they all have a common theme of a "collaborative relationship." I am aware of different conceptualizations of the working alliance and do not suggest that Bordin's definition and the associated measures are superior conceptually or statistically to others. But it has proved to be a highly sound conception that has generated considerable research. Nonetheless, Bedi and Hayes (Chapter 6) note—and in my view do so correctly—that therapists should not impose a singular inflexible view of the alliance (or the working relationship) on their clients. Each client is different, and each alliance takes on the unique qualities of each of the participants. Thus therapist flexibility, the willingness to approach the client where the client is, and the ability to tailor the work to the needs of the client all come in handy in good treatment. This relates to the interpersonal ability that Anderson and Perlman (Chapter 3) call "responsiveness," or the ability of the therapist to shift, change gears, and adapt to the needs of the client at any particular point in therapy. While this ability probably takes time to develop, this is an area where supervision can be extremely valuable, and supervision is valuable in all facets of training and service delivery (Goodyear and Sera, Chapter 9). A good supervisor can help a motivated therapist/supervisee calibrate interventions to achieve what all working alliances seems to entail: the development of a "confident collaborative relationship" that yields good and transformative results for clients.

References

Bordin, E. S. (1979). The generalizability of the psychoanalytic concept of the working alliance. *Psychotherapy: Theory, Research, and Practice, 16*, 252–260. http://dx.doi.org/10.1037/h0085885

Egan, G. (2010). *The skilled helper: A problem management and opportunity development approach to helping* (9th ed.). Pacific Grove, CA: Brooks/Cole Cengage Learning.

Fuertes, J. N., & Williams, L. N. (2017). Client-focused psychotherapy research. *Journal of Counseling Psychology, 64*(4), 369–375. http://dx.doi.org/10.1037/cou0000214.

Hatcher, R. L., & Barends, A. W. (2006). How a return to theory could help alliance research. *Psychotherapy: Theory, Research, Practice, Training, 43*, 292–299. doi:10.1037/0033-3204.43.3.292.

Hill, C. E. (2014). *Helping skills: Facilitating exploration, insight, and action* (4th ed.). Washington, DC: American Psychological Association.

Lambert, M. J. (2013). The efficacy and effectiveness of psychotherapy. In M. J. Lambert (Ed.), *Bergin and Garfield's handbook of psychotherapy and behavior change* (6th ed., pp. 169–218). Hoboken, NJ: Wiley.

Rousmaniere, T. (2016). *Deliberate practice for psychotherapists: A guide to improving clinical effectiveness.* New York: Routledge.

Index

CPSIA information can be obtained
at www.ICGtesting.com
Printed in the USA
BVHW052351060723
666892BV00003B/9